'A timely book which argues that relationship-based care is more important than ever at a time when health care is increasingly fragmented, taskified, deprofessionalised and digitised.'

Professor Trisha Greenhalgh, *University of Oxford*

'An inspiring collection of essays that eloquently diagnoses the dis-ease afflicting contemporary healthcare. And *Finding Meaning in Healthcare* goes beyond diagnosis to offer us the cure – an elegant framework which, applied to every consultation and clinical encounter, will transform the experience of both patients and the practitioners who care for them. Essential reading for anyone who has even an inkling that, for all the spectacular advances of medicine in the scientific era, the practice of healthcare has grievously lost its way.'

Dr Phil Whitaker, *Medical Editor, New Statesman, and author of* What Is a Doctor? – A GP's Prescription for the Future

'Much of general practice and primary care seems to be drowning in anxiety and despondency both for patients and professionals. This book provides some much-needed life rafts!'

Dr Iona Heath, *Past President Royal College of General Practitioners*

I0092091

Finding Meaning in Healthcare

This pioneering book illustrates the ways in which an interpretive or hermeneutic stance can be incorporated into modern healthcare across clinical practice, clinical ethics, education and leadership – and the transformative effects of doing so.

Combining practical case studies and narrative, this book introduces the hermeneutic window, in which meaning making frames clinical and educational decision making. It shows how best practice requires more than clinical knowledge, communication skills and application of evidence based medicine. It is within the hermeneutic window that assumptions, meanings and values are examined, questioned and re-examined. Drawing on a wide range of expertise, the chapters challenge existing assumptions about the essence of healthcare and the role that clinicians play within it.

This book is valuable reading for all healthcare practitioners, particularly GPs, physicians, psychiatrists and psychologists, as well as professions allied to medicine, medical students and other trainees.

Rupal Shah is a GP and medical educator in London. She has published widely in the field of medical education, including *Fighting for the Soul of General Practice – The Algorithm Will See You Now* (2024) and the hermeneutic window series of articles.

Robert Clarke is a retired GP and medical educator who has a longstanding interest in evidence based medicine. He first co-formulated the hermeneutic window to demonstrate that biomedical and humanistic approaches are complementary and has collaborated with Rupal Shah and colleagues in arguing that meaning making is essential in healthcare.

Finding Meaning in Healthcare
Looking Through the Hermeneutic Window

Edited by
Rupal Shah and Robert Clarke

Routledge
Taylor & Francis Group

LONDON AND NEW YORK

Designed cover image: ©David Garaway, used with permission

First published 2026
by Routledge
4 Park Square, Milton Park, Abingdon, Oxon OX14 4RN

and by Routledge
605 Third Avenue, New York, NY 10158

Routledge is an imprint of the Taylor & Francis Group, an informa business

British Library Cataloguing-in-Publication Data
A catalogue record for this book is available from the British Library

ISBN: 9781032853246 (hbk)
ISBN: 9781032832166 (pbk)
ISBN: 9781003517665 (ebk)

DOI: 10.4324/9781003517665

Typeset in Times New Roman
by codeMantra

Contents

Contributors

Editors

Robert Clarke is a retired GP and medical educator who has a longstanding interest in evidence based medicine. He first co-formulated the Four Domain Model to demonstrate that biomedical and humanistic approaches are complementary and has collaborated with Rupal Shah and colleagues in arguing that meaning making is essential in healthcare. ORCID: 0000-0001-8351-5939

Rupal Shah is a GP Partner in London and Associate Dean in London's Professional Development Team (NHS England – Workforce Training and Education). She is the co-author of *Fighting for the Soul of General Practice – The Algorithm Will See You Now*, *Our Mothers Ourselves* and a wide range of peer-reviewed journal articles in the field of medical education, including the Hermeneutic Window series. ORCID: 0000-0001-9079-0971

Chapter authors

Sanjiv Ahluwalia is Head of Anglia Ruskin Medical School. He has been involved in clinical education since 2002 having started as a GP training programme director and most recently has been the Regional Postgraduate Dean for London. His educational work has consisted of managing postgraduate medical training programmes, workforce, and educational transformation with service providers, and developing interprofessional education. His research explores the relationship between clinical education and patient care/outcomes. ORCID: 0000-0002-5830-0853

Sylvie Delacroix is the Inaugural Jeff Price Chair in Digital Law and the Director of the *Centre for data Futures* (King's College London). She is also a visiting professor at the University of Tohoku (Japan). Her research focuses on the role played by habit within ethical agency, the role of humility markers as conversation enablers and the potential inherent in LLMs' participatory interfaces. She also considers bottom-up data empowerment structures and the *social sustainability* of the data ecosystem that makes generative AI possible. The latter work led to the first data trusts pilots worldwide being launched in 2022 in the context of the Data Trusts initiative *www.datatrusts.uk*. Her latest

book *Habitual Ethics?* was published by Bloomsbury in 2022 (*open-access*).
ORCID: 0000-0002-8517-7782.

Jens Foell trained in Germany in Rehabilitation Medicine with special focus
on musculoskeletal disability. He moved to the UK and retrained as GP. He
worked in the deindustrialised areas of Northwest and Northeast England, in
an inner-city practice and as academic GP in London. Currently, he is living in
North Wales. His research interests are the management of pain, mental health
problems and social issues in community settings with special focus on pain
communication. His work activities include substantial service in General Practice alongside educational work as Programme Director for GP Training, Mental
Health Act assessments and GP appraisals. ORCID: 0000-0003-1210-1311

Sabena Jameel has been working as an inner-city GP in Birmingham for 25 years.
She has had senior educational leadership positions in both postgraduate and
undergraduate medical education. Formerly and Associate Dean for GP Education, she is currently Medical Professionalism Lead and Academic Quality Lead
at the University of Birmingham Medical School. Sabena has completed a PhD
at Birmingham University where she looked at enacted Phronesis (practical wisdom) in General Practitioners. This emphasis on values-based practice, character development and professional virtues underpins her approach to teaching
medical professionalism. ORCID: 0000-0002-6654-2596

Jo-Anne Johnson is a leader in medical education, research development, and
clinical practice. As an Associate Professor of Medical Education and Research
Development at Anglia Ruskin University's School of Medicine, she serves as
Head of Undergraduate Medicine and Research Lead, playing a pivotal role in
shaping the future of medical education and training. Clinically, she is a practising paediatrician specialising in Sleep Medicine, and she founded the Paediatric
Ambulatory Sleep Service at East Suffolk and North Essex Foundation Trust,
significantly advancing accessible paediatric sleep care within the region.
ORCID: 0000-0002-9031-7022

Martina Ann Kelly is a Professor of Family Medicine at Cumming School of Medicine, University of Calgary, Alberta, Canada. ORCID: 0000-0002-8763-7092

Emma Ladds is a GP Partner in West Oxfordshire. She is also studying for a PhD
part time at the University of Oxford, exploring the relationships between patients and their GPs in contemporary General Practice and how this influences
health-related behaviours. Prior to starting General Practice training, she completed core surgical training and a Master's degree in Public Health at Harvard
University. ORCID: 0000-0001-9864-7408

John Launer is a GP Educator, Family Therapist and Writer. He is a regular col-
umnist for the BMJ and has written and edited eleven books, including *Narrative Based Practice in Health and Social Care: Conversations Inviting Change '*
and *Reflective Practice in Medicine and Multiprofessional Healthcare*. His current posts include Honorary President of the Association of Narrative Practice

in Healthcare and Visiting Professor at Anglia Ruskin University. ORCID: 0000-0003-3833-9352

Richard Lehman worked as a GP in a small English town for 35 years and later became A Professor of the Shared Understanding of Medicine at the University of Birmingham for three years until he retired completely. He became known for the reviews of the main medical journals he produced every week for 20 years, and he still produces editorials, commentaries and podcasts about evidence based medicine and about the impact of artificial intelligence on medicine and professional values. ORCID: 0000-0003-3259-0239

Marcus Lewis is a GP at the Abbey Medical Centre, Kilburn, London and Training Programme Director for the Royal Free GP Speciality Training Scheme. He is the author of *The Digital Balint: Using AI in Reflective Practice.* ORCID: 0009-0009-0457-6975

Victor Montori is the Robert H. and Susan M. Rewoldt Professor of Medicine at Mayo Clinic. An endocrinologist, health services researcher, and care activist, Dr. Montori is the author of nearly 800 peer-reviewed publications. He is also the 2024–2025 Human Rights and Technology Fellow at Harvard Kennedy School. He is a recognised expert in evidence based medicine, shared decision making, and minimally disruptive medicine. He works in Rochester, Minnesota, at *Mayo Clinic's KER Unit*, to advance person-centred care for patients with diabetes and other chronic conditions. As a care activist, he authored the book *Why We Revolt*, and is leading a movement, a *Patient Revolution*, for Careful and Kind Care for all. ORCID: 0000-0003-0595-2898

Jane Myat has been a GP at the same practice in north London for 27 years. Drawing on her own experiences, knowing that there is more to health than can be delivered in the confines of the consulting room, Jane worked alongside her patients and members of the local community to create a garden in the middle of her group practice. This became known as The Listening Space. Working in and with that space opened up practical possibilities to explore questions: what it is to be well, how we might heal ourselves, each other and the natural world. It also led to meeting others travelling with the same enquiries in the local area.

David Fraile Navarro is a Research Fellow at the Centre for Health Informatics, Australian Institute of Health Innovation at Macquarie University. His work currently centres across the use of novel approaches to health automation and healthcare delivery using Generative AI (such as GPT-4 and related large language models). He is a trained General Practitioner with over seven years of clinical experience in Spain and the UK. He has also previously worked on producing Living Guidelines for COVID-19 and new evidence synthesis methods with Cochrane Australia and Monash University. ORCID: 0000-0002-1108-7071

Austin O'Carroll is an inner-city GP since 1997. The focus of his career has been improving access for communities affected by marginalisation or deprivation to quality primary healthcare, including his formation of Safetynet (2007) which provides

GP services to over 6,000 marginalised patients annually throughout Ireland. He was Dublin HSE Covid Lead for the Homeless Population between 2020 and 2022. He was appointed HSE Clinical Lead for Reviews of Deaths in Homelessness in 2023. He was appointed Chairperson of North Dublin City Drugs Task Force in 2024. He was awarded the 5 Star Doctor Award from Wonca Europe in 2020. He participated in 2016 Paralympics in sailing. ORCID: 0000-0003-3935-5042

Sophie Park is a GP and Professor of Primary Care and Clinical Education at the University of Oxford where she leads the 'Workforce and Learning' Research Group, and is the Director of Undergraduate Studies in Primary Care. Her most recent book *Generalism in Clinical Practice and Education* (UCL Press) examines the importance of generalist approaches across organisation and delivery of care, alongside learning systems. Her current roles include Chair Royal College of General Practice (RCGP) Scientific Foundation Board, Chair Society of Academic Primary Care (SAPC) Education Research Group, Co-Chair NIHR Incubator Clinical Education Research, and Senior Research Fellow at Harris Manchester College. She is committed to patient partnership in her clinical and academic roles, advocating for the inclusion of patient and public within clinical education research and practice. ORCID: 0000-0002-1521-2052

Jane Riddiford has a wealth of experience in creating the conditions for good community. Her work has involved growing an urban forest in Auckland, working with story, whether that be in street theatre or in circles in many different places. Jane co-founded the charity, Global Generation in London, bringing environmental education to young people, their families and the local community. In her book, *Learning to Lead Together: An Ecological and Community Approach*, Jane writes about her experience of how collaborative, participatory and practical enquiry has supported much of the community work she has done. Jane has a strong belief in the value of collaborative, participatory and practical enquiry. She has returned to her native New Zealand and co-founded Ruamāhanga Farm Foundation, a community-oriented wetland and riparian forest restoration project

Melissa Sayer is a GP Partner and Educator in East London; and Associate Dean in London's Professional Development Team (NHS England – Workforce Training and Education).

John Spicer is a GP is South London and a Teacher of Clinical Ethics and Law in various Universities and postgraduate areas. He has written widely on medical ethics, particularly with reference to primary care and the medical humanities. ORCID: 0000-0002-1700-4038

Sami Timimi is a Consultant Child and Adolescent Psychiatrist in the National Health Service in Lincolnshire, UK. He writes from a critical psychiatry perspective on topics relating to mental health and childhood and has published over 140 articles in mainstream medical, educational, and sociological journals. He has written 40 book chapters, mainly in academic books, on subjects related to critical psychiatry, childhood, psychotherapy, depression, behavioural problems, and cross-cultural psychiatry. He has authored seven books, including *Naughty Boys: Anti-Social Behaviour, ADHD and the Role of Culture*, co-edited four books, including, with Carl Cohen, *Liberatory Psychiatry: Philosophy, Politics and Mental Health*, and co-authored two others, including, with Neil Gardiner and Brian McCabe, *The Myth of Autism: Medicalising Men's and Boys' Social and Emotional Competence*. His latest book, *Searching for Normal*, will be published in March 2025. ORCID: 0000-0001-5768-2231

Louise Younie is a General Practitioner and Professor of Medical Education at Queen Mary University of London where she leads on faculty development, innovation and flourishing. She has extensive experience with creative enquiry methodologies in medical education for humanising medicine, professional identity formation and human flourishing. She is the co-chair of the *Royal College of GPs Creative Health Special Interest Group* (SIG). She is a National Teaching Fellow (2022) and holds a Principal Fellowship of the Higher Education Academy. Perhaps her greatest learning has been through her journey in 2014 as a cancer patient. ORCID: 0000-0003-3412-993X

Paquita de Zulueta worked for 38 years as an inner-city, London-based GP and during this time developed a special interest and expertise in mental health, migrant health, clinical ethics, medical education, and professional wellbeing and development. She is an honorary senior lecturer at Imperial College, an integrative cognitive behavioural therapist (CBT) and a qualified coach and mentor. Paquita teaches, researches and writes about clinical ethics, leadership and compassion in healthcare. She is a trustee of the Institute of Medical Ethics and a member of the RCGP ethics committee. Paquita is the chair of the Human Values in Healthcare Forum, a charity whose key aim is to rehumanise healthcare. ORCID: 0000-0002-5260-8830

Foreword

I find asymptotic lines fascinating. Parallel ones never meet. Intersecting ones do so for an instant only to never meet again. An asymptotic line constantly approaches another line. The space between them narrows as they get closer till they almost touch; beyond then, they get closer still.

This is the space between the fingertips of each of the two distinct hands that Rodin sculpted to form his Cathedral. This is the space, between patient and clinician, within which they come to understand how to advance the situation of the patient, and, in doing so, they get closer. This is the space to which they return to recover from disappointment and to celebrate discoveries, alleviations, improvements, and, in doing so, they get closer.

To this space they arrive, unhurriedly. And here it is where the situation, because of what they do in proximity, becomes clearer, more manageable. Here is where patients remember that their lives matter, where clinicians remember their care matters. This is where they are close enough to notice what is the matter, but also where it is possible to form a sensible response. This is the space of responsiveness, of hope. The space of meaning making. The space of care.

Industrialised healthcare processes people, delivering diagnoses and treatments quickly and from afar. Too far to notice the patient situation in high definition, the clinician moves on to the next one, gone too fast to find out whether the response was adequate, pertinent, and desirable to this person. Lines that should be asymptotic instead only manage to intersect and then drift meaninglessly away, leaving both unable to tell a story of care.

As it becomes digital, industrialised healthcare confuses the problems of care with problems of information, shifting capabilities from processing patients to processing their data. Data collection, retrieval, organisation, analysis, and display displace and replace the work of making sense of each patient's troubling situation. Drowned in data, but thirsty for meaning, clinicians cannot match the performance of AI systems, systems that can feign empathy yet depart unchanged from their encounters with suffering. With their care-mission corrupted, info-care organisations can operate at scales of speed and reach that are only possible by avoiding the human asymptote.

Although information is often a helpful tool, the problem of care is not a problem of information. To have data about me, is not the same as understanding my situation; to offer the right answer about what to do for people like me is often not the same as figuring out with me how we are going to advance my situation. The problem of care, particularly when there is no right answer, demands that patients and clinicians craft together a useful story, one that makes the situation less troubling, one that points at and moves us towards the way forward, one that reintegrates, restores, reweaves broken life tapestries. It is in this space of co-creation, in the asymptote, that patients and clinicians develop and hold meaning.

A powerful movement seeks to turn away from the digital industrialisation of healthcare and towards careful and kind care for everyone. This movement, a patient revolution, calls for recognising that only people can care. And that people can only care at human scale and speed. And that healthcare must create conditions for care to happen in proximity, in closeness, where the lines nearly abut, where the fingertips almost touch.

Let this book fuel that movement for care to ensure that patients and clinicians find each other where time deepens, and care happens: in the asymptote where meaning is made.

Victor Montori, MD

1 An introduction to the Four Domain Model

Robert Clarke and Rupal Shah

As clinicians, we are practising in an era in which individualised care is more vital than ever, given the fragmentation within healthcare systems, the sheer number of interventions on offer, defensive practice and the increasingly remote nature of patient-clinician encounters. We can't offer this individualised care unless we try to understand our patients' experience of illness and what it means to them; what matters most to them; and simultaneously understand our own motivations and emotions during these interactions. For this to be possible, we need to hone our interpretive ability; this is the reason we proposed a model that incorporates interpretation and finding meaning through context (hermeneutics) (Shah et al., 2020, 2021, 2022, 2022a, 2022b, 2022c, 2023). In this book, we will expand on what is involved in creating meaning through context, not only in the consultation, but also in medical education, when adopting technology such as artificial intelligence (AI) and what difference finding meaning might make to us as practitioners within the healthcare system.

The biopsychosocial model of illness (Engel, 1977) has been accepted within mainstream clinical practice for almost 50 years, and with it, an acknowledgement of the importance of gathering information about the social and psychological contexts of our patients. However, the model has been understood and implemented by clinicians in different ways, often with a focus on gathering data, rather than responding to the individual circumstances and life worlds of patients.

Concurrently, evidence based medicine has become firmly established within healthcare over recent decades, leading to the creation of clinical guidelines that we are advised to interpret according to the individual circumstances of our patients. Yet, there has been little advice about how to integrate these different paradigms (Clarke & Croft, 1998) in a context where medicolegal fears and a culture of standardisation discourage deviation from rules. In fact, relational care, predicated on connection between practitioners and patients, seems to have become significantly eroded, particularly after the COVID-19 pandemic, with 'care' increasingly being experienced as anonymous, remote and generic. Perhaps it isn't surprising therefore that there has been, in tandem, a huge attrition of practitioners from the NHS.

In this book, we will attempt to take a step beyond the biopsychosocial, by explaining how the incorporation of meaning making into the consultation and more broadly into clinical practice and even into creation of healthcare policy might help to inject joy into our work.

DOI: 10.4324/9781003517665-1

The Four Domain Model

The Four Domain Model (Shah et al., 2020) is intended to describe the skills and attributes that contribute to whole person care. It is represented as a two-by-two table with four separate but related domains (see Figure 1.1). The first column is labelled biomedical and is supported by the natural sciences, while the second column is labelled humanistic and has its foundation within the social sciences. Window 1 consists of clinical skills, such as history taking and physical examination of different systems, underpinned by knowledge, including an awareness of current guidelines.

The second window directly above this, evidence based practice, represents the application of such knowledge and skills to a specific patient in a specific context, rather than being based on a population in a clinical trial. This usually entails an increase in complexity and is frequently also accompanied by an increase in uncertainty because the 'right' answer for an individual patient may not be certain, even in the face of clear evidence from the scientific literature.

Within the humanistic column, communication skills (window 3) go beyond basic history taking to include some of the skills of person-centred consulting, for example, eliciting a patient's ideas and concerns about their symptoms and using patient expectations as a basis for negotiating a shared management plan.

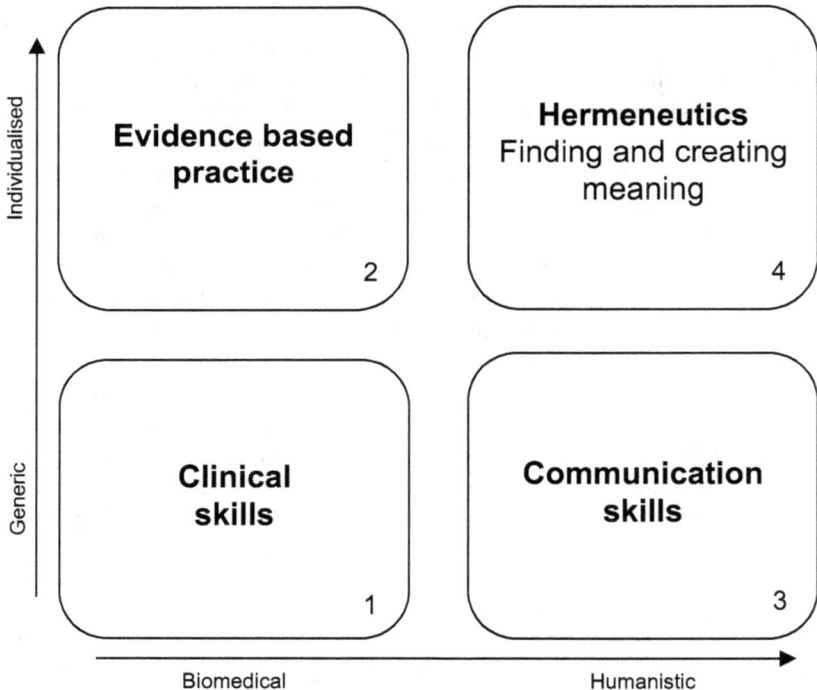

Figure 1.1 The Four Domain Model (Shah et al., 2020).

Finally, we reach the hermeneutic window (window 4) where assumptions, meanings and roles are interpreted in a way which is particular to the individual. This is often the area of greatest complexity and uncertainty, where questions about what it means to be a healthcare professional are asked and relationships with individual patients are examined. It entails reflective practice and the exploration of values and beliefs. What are the assumptions, biases and judgements that inform clinical decision making? What are the external influences on the consultation – for example, performance incentive schemes, external quality regulators, fear of litigation and time pressures? This is also where validation of a patient's experience ('doctor as witness') is important (Heath, 2018); where a practitioner may trigger a new insight, with a 'catalytic intervention' (Heron, 2001); or may help a patient to move on from a stuck autobiographical narrative (Launer, 2008). Central to this is a view of individuals as having both agency and creative capacity (Reeve, 2010), and an active effort on the part of the clinician to redress narrative power imbalance (see also Chapter 7). A hermeneutic gaze can be equally powerful in supporting, challenging and transforming both clinicians and patients.

An underlying theme in every chapter in this book is that finding meaning in healthcare is all about how you position yourself as a practitioner: how you see your role. Many people reading this will already be training or working as hermeneutic practitioners and would rather view this approach as underpinning the other three domains and not an adjunct – in which case they may find the alternative model in Figure 1.2 appealing (Clarke, 2025).

However, we see the main purpose of a model as being simply to draw attention to something important. This model in Figure 1.2 could be taken to assume that the practitioner is already working in a hermeneutic way and does not challenge us to consider either what this means or the frequently neglected implications in terms of values, beliefs, training and practice, which are explored in this book. Most importantly, critics of a meaning-based approach to healthcare may imply that this is something soft and fluffy that can easily be dismissed. Our purpose in writing this book is to demonstrate that meaning making is an essential complement to, not

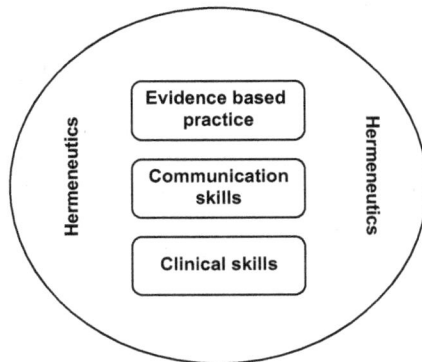

Figure 1.2 An Alternative Model (Clarke, 2025).

a replacement for excellent clinical care and evidence based medicine: hence, we put it alongside evidence based practice in Figure 1.1. We therefore invite you to consider the Four Domain Model and invite even those who have embraced this approach to explore further the hermeneutic window.

Finding and creating meaning in a specific context

Within the biopsychosocial frame, we might ask questions about someone's social context and their mental health, but doing this alone might not enable us to understand the meaning behind what has been said or equip us to respond to suffering. When a clinician meets a patient who is suffering, it isn't usually articulated in those terms. Consider the frail 85 year old who comes in with non-specific chest pain but whose mortality is a third presence in the room, where the untellable heart of the consultation is, 'I am frightened that I am dying. I don't know how to deal with this'; or the 25-year-old woman with personality disorder who comes in about her chronic pain and nobody mentions that it might be related to the sexual abuse she was subject to as a child; the woman with memory loss who feels her life unravelling around her; the child with abdominal pain whose parents are always fighting because of financial insecurity.

It appears to us that suffering is not permissible within our current healthcare paradigm. As clinicians, we are encouraged to categorise it into something that is easier to get a handle on, to reduce and define. So, within the confines of a time-pressured consultation, the 85-year-old man might be referred to a rapid access chest pain clinic. The 25 year old might be prescribed a painkiller and signed off work. The woman with memory loss could be referred to a memory clinic. The child with abdominal pain might have blood tests or an ultrasound. We tend to concentrate on the label on the tin and assume it reflects what is contained inside.

The tension between guidelines and person-centred care

We live in a world where we have become accustomed to breaking things down into their component parts and then outsourcing them. This applies to society in general and is not a phenomenon limited to healthcare. However, a manifestation of this type of thinking in clinical practice is a proliferation of pathways, algorithms, targets and measurements: what Don Berwick has called 'era 2 medicine' (Berwick, 2016). As clinicians, we are encouraged to provide 'holistic patient-centred care'; yet, the reality is that all our guidelines are disease focussed and are predicated on categorisation, often aided by triage tools. Once a category has been chosen, the pathway must be followed, regardless of the person behind the category and their story. There is a fundamental assumption that causality is linear and that outcomes can be predicted, which is not congruent with the lived human experience of illness. Here is an example:

Mr M is an 84 year old man who lives with his 82 year old wife, Mrs M. They have two grown up daughters, only one of whom still lives nearby.

Mrs M approaches her GP with concerns that Mr M might be developing dementia – he is becoming more forgetful and is still applying for consultancy work, though he hasn't been in formal employment for more than ten years, when he finally retired from his career in the diplomatic service. She wonders whether he should be referred to the memory clinic. The GP asks Mrs M more about how she and her daughters are managing and also about the effect that a diagnosis of dementia would have on her husband, explaining the sources of support that such a diagnosis would give them access to. On reflection, Mrs M thinks that a diagnosis of dementia would be likely to damage Mr M's self-confidence and sense of self. She wonders whether getting him help to write his memoirs might give him a renewed sense of purpose and might be better than pursuing a medical route at this stage. The GP is supportive but advises that blood tests to exclude reversible causes of memory loss could be useful. Mrs M agrees to discuss the conversation they have had with Mr M and with her daughters.

In this case, the GP has been able to integrate her biomedical knowledge with an exploration of what memory loss means for both Mr and Mrs M in their own particular situation, recognising that usually, disease impacts not only on the index patient but also on their family and social networks. She has explained the benefits and limitations of a diagnosis of dementia and offered the potential 'easy win' of screening for (and treating) evidence based, reversible causes of memory loss. In this way, she has successfully integrated windows 2 and 4 – the individualised application of the biomedical with uncovering meaning for the patient and their family. In doing so, she has avoided a referral which might be costly – not only in monetary terms. There is an acceptance by the GP that life is unpredictable and that we may not have ultimate control over outcome but can only hope to influence process, so that we interpret the evidence base in a way that takes into account the lived experience and values of our patients. A consequence of this type of practice is that the relationship between the clinician and patient is strengthened, bringing meaning to the practitioner and perhaps serving to reduce burn out.

In order to reframe healthcare so that people are treated as individuals and that the relationship between practitioner and patient is properly valued, we propose that window 4 in our model – finding and creating meaning – is essential. We are so caught up with the need to acquire knowledge that there is a danger that the skills needed to navigate window 4 and to integrate it with the other domains are overlooked as 'soft skills' that are optional, only to be deployed if the clinician has time – and which are not as important as the skills needed to execute the other domains. We argue that finding and creating meaning is in no way 'soft.' Arguably, it is much easier to follow a guideline than to weigh up medical information within the context of the lived experience of the patient and their family. Yet, these are essential skills if we want a person-centred, sustainable healthcare system that is founded on trust. Figure 1.3 opens up the hermeneutic window to show what might be located within it.

Practitioner as witness
Practitioner's biographical function
Practitioner's use of self

Intuition in partnership with evidence
How do I sense this?
How do I use the different ways of knowing?

Hermeneutic window

Narrative practice
Emotional engagement and connection
Authenticity and curiosity
Relational ethical framework

Exploring professionalism
What is my role here?
What assumptions am I making?
How do my own experiences affect the interaction?

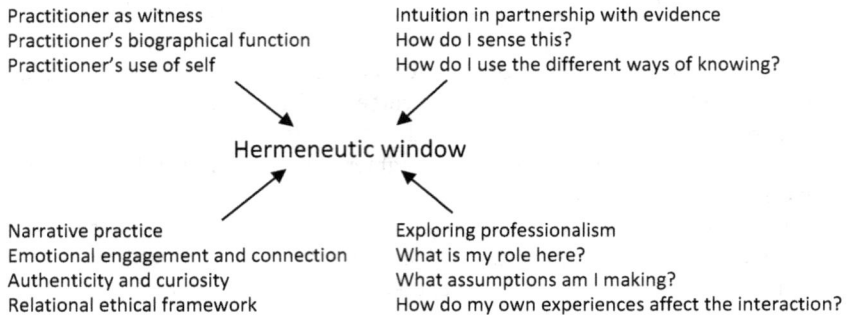

Figure 1.3 Opening Up the Hermeneutic Window (Shah et al., 2021).

Our intention in publishing this book is to articulate the value and need for the integration of the biomedical with hermeneutics, to enable person-centred decision making that is sustainable, meaningful and that enhances the creative capacity of patients (Reeve, 2010). The chapters in the book consider meaning making from a variety of angles: from individual interactions in different contexts (e.g. complex multimorbidity, mental health and chronic pain); to the role of meaning making in education and ethics; in addressing social justice; and how it might help practitioners to flourish. Looking to the future, Marcus Lewis et al. consider how implementation of AI might either promote or shut down meaning making. As we enter a new era of medicine in which these technologies will become ever more dominant, we must not lose sight of medicine as a human enterprise in which creating meaning for ourselves and our patients is integral.

References

Berwick, D. (2016). Era 3 for medicine and health care. *Journal of the American Medical Association, 315*(13), 1329–1330.

Clarke, R. (2025). *Hermeneutic practice: An alternative model.* Diagram.

Clarke, R., & Croft, P. (1998). *Critical reading for the reflective practitioner.* Butterworth Heinemann.

Engel, G. (1977). The need for a new medical model: A challenge for biomedicine. *Science, 196*(4286), 129–136.

Heath, I. (2018). *Matters of life and death: Key writings.* Routledge.

Heron, J. (2001). *Helping the client: A creative practical guide.* Sage Publications.

Launer, J. (2008). Conversations inviting change. *Postgraduate Medical Journal, 84*(987), 4–5.

Reeve, J. (2010). Interpretive medicine: Supporting generalism in a changing primary care world. *Occasional Paper (Royal College of General Practitioners), 88,* 1–20.

Shah, R., Clarke, R., Ahluwalia, S., & Launer, J. (2020). Finding meaning in the consultation: Introducing the hermeneutic window. *British Journal of General Practice, 70*(699), 502–503.

Shah, R., Clarke, R., Ahluwalia, S., & Launer, J. (2021). Finding meaning in the consultation: Working in the hermeneutic window. *British Journal of General Practice, 71*(707), 282–283.

Shah, R., Clarke, R., Ahluwalia, S., & Launer, J. (2022). Finding meaning in the consultation: Supporting the hermeneutic window in practice. *British Journal of General Practice*, *72*(715), 83–84. https://doi.org/10.3399/bjgp22X718493

Shah, R., Clarke, R., Ahluwalia, S., & Launer, J. (2022a). Finding meaning in medical education–how the hermeneutic window can help primary care educators. *Education for Primary Care*, *33*(5), 308–311.

Shah, R., Clarke, R., Ahluwalia, S., & Launer, J. (2022b). Finding meaning in the hidden curriculum–the use of the hermeneutic window in medical education. *Education for Primary Care*, *33*(3), 132–136.

Shah, R., Clarke, R., Ahluwalia, S., & Launer, J. (2022c). Finding meaning, locating hope. *British Journal of General Practice*, *72*(723), 488–489. https://doi.org/10.3399/bjgp22X720845

Shah, R., Clarke, R., Ahluwalia, S., Launer, J., & Spicer, J. (2023). Measuring meaning. *British Journal of General Practice*, *73*(730), 226–227. https://doi.org/10.3399/bjgp23x732813

2 A history of hermeneutics

Emma Ladds

The man before me paused, thinking. 'You know, it's funny, isn't it,' he began, 'I've never really thought about why I don't get breathless at work. And I walk miles around the golf-course in all weathers and it never seems to trouble me.'

I said nothing. We had been chatting for a good 20 minutes now. My afternoon clinic was spiralling out of control. I had heard a lot about his breathlessness, how he had to pause at the top of the stairs, slightly dizzy and force air into his lungs. He was sure the extra weight he was carrying – the result of his irritable bowel syndrome – didn't help. 'I'm just so afraid of being caught short in a field if I take the dog out. It's so embarrassing, doctor,' he'd explained.

I'd heard about his contentious divorce, financial fears and the stress associated with moving in with his sister, 'She doesn't mean to nag. Her heart's in the right place and I don't really listen anyway after a couple of glasses of wine.' I'd heard about his mother's bowel cancer and the fearful memory of his father's vascular dementia. In return, I had explained the many investigations he had been through that made heart or lung disease, cancer, dementia or other organic pathology unlikely. 'Do you know, I've been wondering if some of this might be stress,' he interjected.

The process of interpretation, of making sense of human experience, is a fundamental human endeavour. Coming from the ancient Greek *hermeneuein* (to utter, explain, translate) (OED, 2023), the term 'hermeneutics' has been applied to the process of understanding written or spoken communication. For ancient Greek philosophers, recorded words were the expressions of inner thoughts that required interpretation in order to be fully understood.

Initially, 'hermeneutics' referred to the interpretation of divine messages. Such missives were invariably ambiguous, to the point of irrationality and were therefore considered to be unintelligible to all but a 'divine hermeneut' who could interpret their meaning and authenticity. In Greek mythology, this role was assumed by Hermes, the winged, eloquent trickster, who acted as the 'messenger of the Gods.' Mediating between Gods and men, he allegedly invented speech and language and used the ambiguous power of words and signs to generate unease in their recipients (Hoy, 1982).

Although mythical, Hermes is nevertheless a useful symbol. As Heidegger points out, as the messenger of the Gods, Hermes brings, 'fateful tidings' – messages of great import or significance for their receiver (Heidegger, 1971). In so doing, he

DOI: 10.4324/9781003517665-2

must both transmit such missives effectively, whilst also interpreting their meaning for the recipient. As Walter Otto points out, Hermes enjoys sudden flashes of inspiration (Otto, 1979), which are morally neutral, with meaning and relevance determined by the recipient.

But what does Hermes have to do with a middle-aged, breathless man describing his contentious divorce and alcoholic tendencies to his GP? The answer is that his role chimes with a fundamental part of my own role as a GP – that of interpretation of physical symptoms in the context of narrative.

Hermeneutic philosophers have argued that interpretation is not just something we do, but something we *are*. As Gadamer explains, 'We bring our whole selves to the act of interpretation – our experiences, emotions, and biases shape our understanding' (Gadamer, 1989). Human knowing always involves interpretation – it is not just about facts or information but how we determine and understand the whole meaning behind them. Gradually, focus has moved to the tools humans possess to enable this interpretation, including language and symbolism, history and experience, personal reflection and socio-cultural analysis.

Language and history

Arguments about language, its origin, purpose and intellectual interpretation, have existed for millennia. There is no doubt about the power of words and the role they play in helping us discover the truth about ourselves and the world we inhabit. For some philosophers such as Schleiermacher, thought only happens because of language, with meaning emerging in a continual circle between a part and the whole. One can only infer meaning by considering the relation between the two.

Schleiermacher's approach initiated a tradition, later continued by Dilthey, Husserl, Heidegger, Gadamer and others, which emphasised the relational aspect of hermeneutics. Underlying influences such as context, intention and socio-cultural practices must be considered in order to access the full meaning of language. This can be illustrated by considering the old adage, 'Sticks and stones may break my bones, but words can never hurt me,' designed to help children withstand the torture of bullying. Even as they say it, parents know it to be a lie; yet, it has been in common usage for more than 150 years. Every adult knows 'sticks and stones' are a symbolic representation of physical violence and that the saying illustrates the power of self-belief as a way to stave off the verbal harm inflicted by bullies. Every child who has been the subject of hurtful taunts knows the literal meaninglessness of the phrase. Gradually however, it may gain relevance as they develop an appreciation for the underlying cultural significance and come to see it as an idealistic illustration of a world they would like for their own children. Words refer to objects, events and ideas; they aid learning and help us establish our place in the world and how we relate to it. However, imagery, metaphor and symbolism rely on a socio-cultural understanding that surpasses literality. With reference to the saying, over time, we integrate moral understanding, symbolic imagery, metaphor, a biological and cultural desire to protect our own genetic offspring, alongside a range of other insights to form a holistic meaning for the phrase and the ambiguity of its message.

In time, the concept of relationality was developed by Heidegger into the 'hermeneutic circle,' whereby a holistic reality is situated in the detailed experience of an individual's everyday experience, with a continual, cyclical movement and integration between the two (Heidegger, 1962). This led to the notion that reality can only be generated *through* our engagement with the world (Zimmermann, 2015). Heidegger's famous example is a hammer, which is perceived as 'being in the world,' i.e. a part of our project of hanging a picture. However, it is only when the hammer breaks that we consider it as an abstract object separate from its role in hanging the picture (Heidegger, 1962).

For Heidegger, there are two crucial elements involved in this cultural perception: language and history. As discussed above, language plays a crucial role in meaning making but for Heidegger it is something greater still. 'Language is the house of being,' he claims, 'in its home, man dwells' (Heidegger, 1978). In other words, it is language that enables us to have a world at all (p. 217).

A similar significance is applied to the temporal, historical nature of our existence. How do we connect with the norms and traditions that allow us to form an idea of what a hammer's 'being in the world' means? For Heidegger, the answer is history. It is only through these historical links that we can meaningfully interpret the present.

For my breathless patient, a discussion about his symptoms was contingent on a linguistic appreciation of the word 'breathing.' 'Breathe,' 'inhale,' 'wheeze' – all impart a particular, cultural meaning that would have been absent were the words not there to describe them. He and I were both aware of the sense of fear that 'breathlessness' conveys. Does it mean lung cancer, tuberculosis or a panic attack? His symptoms gained cultural relevance from historical photographs of iron lungs and consumptives; the bleak irony of old 'Joe the Camel' cigarette advertisements, laced with a 'modern' understanding of the risks; and a recognition that physical panic in today's world often represents a sense of stress, overwhelm, a need for change. As Gadamer would later describe in his famous book *Truth and Method*, our awareness comes about because of the effect history has on our perception and of the world (Gadamer, 1989).

Challenges for hermeneutics

Gadamer did not believe that understanding happened in isolation. Rather, he saw it as emerging through multiple processes of participation. Our place in history allows us to engage with traditions, perspectives and ideas from the past; our senses enable a daily engagement with language and metaphor, symbolism and artistic insights; and our interactions and conversations with others and everyday activities allow us to take part in continuous negotiations and mediations to integrate the above impressions into a complete, recognisable picture.

One challenge to this process is that of relativism. How do I know I am not just interpreting texts, conversations, or cultural traditions to align with my own thoughts and views of the world? How do I know my interpretation that my breathless patient IS anxious is the correct one? For E.D. Hirsch, the American educator and literary critic who was sceptical of relativism, the 'correct' interpretation was the one that aligned with the original author's intended meaning (Hirsch, 1967). However, for Ricoeur, who opposed Hirsch's criticism, subjective, personal choice and ethical values play essential roles in the construction of meaning. He argued that when we are trying to devise 'meaning,' we are always seeking for the richest possible interpretation of the world. Therefore, different individuals may offer deeper insights, enhanced by approaches from the arts and humanities alongside critical reflection and a well-developed imagination (Pellauer & Dauenhauer, 2022).

Hermeneutics in science and medicine

The Scientific Revolution of the sixteenth and seventeenth centuries saw a transformation in our approach towards knowledge, dominated by a move towards scientific objectivism. Rejecting the ancient Greek traditions that included insights from philosophy and the arts in our quest for knowledge, instinct gave way to abstract reasoning; a quantitative outlook superceded the qualitative; nature came to be seen as explicable by reducing it down to the sum of its parts, rather than acknowledging the inherent uncertainty in any complex system; and a rational empirical approach took hold, emphasising the 'how' at the expense of the 'why.' Underpinned by the literal Latin translation of their craft – *'scientia'* meaning *'knowledge'* – scientists came to be seen as those who *'knew'* truth and facts, whilst others merely believed (Zimmermann, 2015).

This led to the perception that adopting scientific empiricism leads to 'objective truth' – the highest form of knowledge. This worldview, which took hold in the eighteenth and nineteenth centuries has subsequently dominated much of our approach towards knowledge. Not only does it promote the primacy of a positivist outlook, i.e. there *is* an objective truth or fact out there to be discovered, but it also ignores the contribution of human factors. Lippman has described how 'people live in the same world, but they think and feel in different ones' (Lippmann, 1922). He argued that the size, speed and complexity of the 'whole environment' of reality lead individuals to create their own abridged, subjective and biased mental imagery of the world (pseudo-environment) that has meaning for them – a form of social constructionism. Humans thus exist within their own, constructed reality that incorporates their socio-cultural context and 'objective' facts are always considered within that framework. Feyerabend extrapolated this to propose that scientific experimentation is never unbiased but always *'theory-laden'* (Feyerabend, 1975), i.e. scientists approach their quest for 'the truth' through their own socio-culturally determined view of the world.

Within medicine, the move towards rationalism has had widespread consequences. An empirical approach to disease and the diagnostic and therapeutic developments this enabled have resulted in numerous health benefits for individuals and the population as a whole. Gone are the days when General Practitioners (GPs) 'knew so little and understood so little'; when a splodge of blood coughed onto a handkerchief meant a case of tuberculosis, or when faced with a case of pneumonia the GP was 'forced to stand by helpless and watch a strapping young man die in six days without being able to influence the disease in the slightest' (Elder, 1964). Instead, the introduction of penicillin and subsequent rollout of mass vaccination led the wave of therapeutic options that turned doctors from the familiar role of guide, philosopher and friend into biomedical scientists, equipped with an impressive armoury of modern 'cures.' The infant mortality rate fell from around 36 in 1,000 in the 1950s to 8 in 1,000 in 1990; and the 400–500 per 100,000 women who died in pregnancy prior to 1930 reduced to 10 in 100,000 in 1990 (Loudon et al., 1998). The doctor's gaze becomes profoundly focused on the physical, with a pejorative stigmatisation of the psychological. For example, Taylor, a GP writing in 1954, argued that, 'the better the doctor, the less often does he diagnose neurosis' (Taylor, 1954).

Although the Balint method in general practice and the patient-centred medicine movement of the 1990s continued to highlight the importance of the doctor-patient relationship and holistic care, the evidence based medicine (EBM) movement of the 1990s reinvigorated the positivist approach to medicine. This approach, facilitated by the introduction of the computer with its potential for quantitative monitoring and algorithmic care, highlighted the importance of using the 'best' evidence to guide decisions around medical management (Sackett et al., 1996). Professional judgement, communities of practice and intuition were cast aside in favour of a quest for the 'highest' form of empirical evidence. Different types of scientific studies were deemed to produce a rank of knowledge that strove to reach a positivist truth. Although there is no universally accepted hierarchy (Siegfried, 2017), case studies traditionally occupy the lowest rank as they are concerned with an in-depth knowledge of the particular, whilst systemic reviews and meta-analyses are valued for their many participants and thus are located towards the top.

Despite its positive contribution to health outcomes – between 1980 and 2013, for example, UK mortality from cardiovascular disease has declined by 68% (Bhatnagar et al., 2016) – the EBM movement has been criticised for its overly reductionist outlook. Evidence hierarchies prioritise quantitative metrics over qualitative. Whilst attractive to policy makers and those in control of the healthcare budget, such a focus directs both the physician and system towards numbers rather than values. Although Sackett, the founder of EBM, envisaged it as the 'judicious use of current best evidence in making decisions about the care of individual patients,' which involved 'integrating individual clinical expertise with the best available external clinical evidence from systematic reviews' (Sackett et al., 1996), in reality, external evidence usually trumps individual clinical expertise these days. Sackett envisaged individual clinical expertise as that acquired through clinical practice and experience, *reflected in many ways but especially in more effective and efficient diagnosis and in the more thoughtful identification and compassionate use of individual patients' predicaments, rights, and preferences in making clinical decisions about their care* (Sackett et al., 1996). Importantly, the patient should be involved in determining the values that underpin decisions made about them.

Shah and Clarke et al. have proposed a Four Domain Model to consider the combination of four 'windows': clinical knowledge and skill; evidence based practice; communication skills and hermeneutics (see Figure 2.1). Successfully

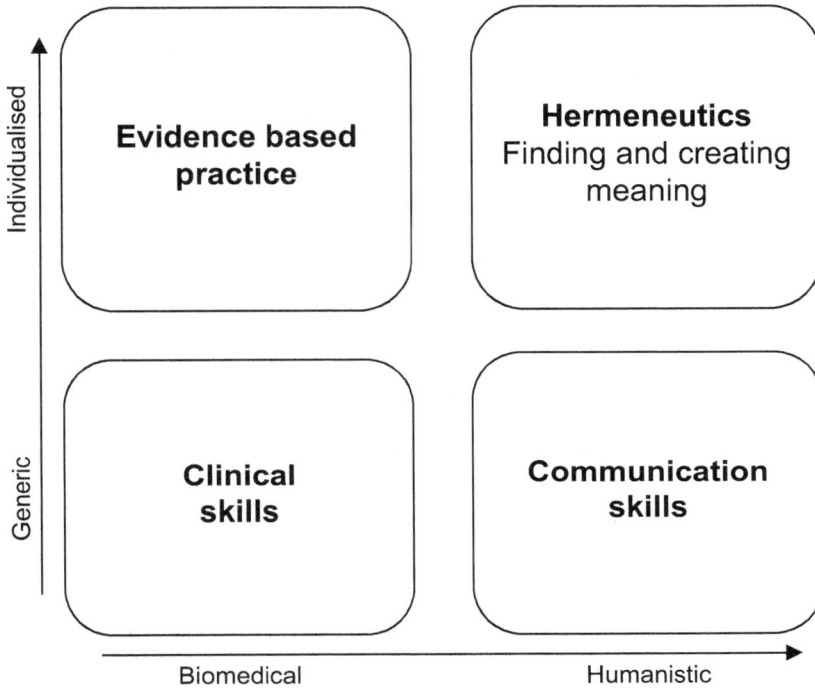

Figure 2.1 The Four Domain Model, Introducing the Hermeneutic Window (Shah et al., 2021).

integrating the first three elements can enable a person-centred application of skills and knowledge for a particular individual in a specific context. However, the most challenging window is the hermeneutic, which requires a shared interpretation of assumptions, meanings and roles particular to the patient and doctor in that moment. It is here that a web of meanings can emerge through reflective practice with a wealth of insightful, agentic and creative effects (Shah et al., 2021). Throughout this book, we will contend that meaning making is integral to applied EBM and is not an 'optional extra.'

In recent years, performative incentivisation schemes that are underpinned by digital data capture have made it more challenging for clinicians to deploy professional judgement. For example, if I add a code to my breathless patient's electronic record to note the fact that he is breathless, I will be endlessly prompted to refer him for spirometry assessment (for which my local Primary Care Network will receive a payment); enter his weight – to determine if he is eligible for a similarly incentivised weight management referral; or consider his smoking status, whether he needs a chest x-ray, and numerous other processes that may have little relevance to the man before me.

This neoliberal paradigm, stemming from Thatcher's introduction of free market principles and the centralisation programme of the New Labour movement, has significantly influenced conceptualisations of healthcare. It is no longer sufficient to care for the individual patient, isolated from their population cohort – rather, there is an implication that they are a number and have to be considered as such. Illness, within such a framework, must be viewed at the population level as much as at the individual level. In a resource-constrained system, after I have asked my patient about his smoking status and weight, referred him for spirometry, a chest x-ray and a weight management programme, I have little time, if any, to ask him about himself.

In this drive for efficiency, ticking all my boxes and optimising all my numbers would never allow me near the golf course that offers him a reprieve of his symptoms. I would never feel his embarrassment at having to squat in a field or hear about the acrimonious encounters with his soon-to-be-ex-wife. I would never 'meet' his bossy sister or understand how alcohol helps him to escape her admonitions. In a system focused on measurable activity, where *doing* matters, compassion and human connection have little place.

And yet, it is *only* through such connection and care that meaning arises. Only by listening will that moment of intimacy arise. A sentence so short you can count the words, 'I've been wondering if it might be stress.' And in that moment, that flash of insight, acknowledgement and acceptance offers a multitude of true efficiencies even if the consultation itself took longer. The extra time spent means I can use our connection to explain the surge of adrenaline that courses through the body in times of stress, stimulating bowels and tensing muscles. I can show him the hunched posture of anxiety that restricts the intercostal muscles and prevents deep breaths, help him feel the quickening heart rate and rapid breaths of a human preparing for 'fight or flight.' It will be a path that avoids unnecessary investigations and costly scans; that over time reduces his dependence on doctors and counsellors and offers him more agency. Longer appointments in which attention to hermeneutics is central might well increase overall system efficiency.

Conclusion

Human beings are complex and challenging. We are meaning-makers who rely on integrating multiple perspectives to make sense of our world, our place within it and ourselves. Hermeneutics pervades all aspects and disciplines of human life and philosophers and scientists across the ages have struggled to come to terms with how we pursue this quest for knowledge and truth. Truly meaningful interpretation relies on a balance of perceptions and socio-cultural influences. These are personal and value-laden and cannot be reduced to a mere number, no matter how large it may be.

References

Bhatnagar, P., Wickramasinghe, K., Wilkins, E., & Townsend, N. (2016). Trends in the epidemiology of cardiovascular disease in the UK. *Heart, 102*(24), 1945–1952.

Elder, H. (1964). Forty years in general practice. *The Journal of the College of General Practitioners, 7*(3), 328.

Feyerabend, P. (1975). *Against method: Outline of an anarchistic theory of knowledge.* New Left Books.

Gadamer, H- G. (1989). *Truth and method.* A&C Black.

Heidegger, M. (1962). *Being and time.* Blackwell.

Heidegger, M. (1971). *On the way to language*. Harper & Row.

Heidegger, M. (1978). Letter on humanism. In D. F. Krell (Ed.), *Basic writings* (pp. 189–242). Routledge.

Hirsch, E. D. (1967). *Validity in interpretation*. Yale University Press.

Hoy, D. (1982). *The critical circle*. University of California Press.

Lippmann, W. (1922). *Public opinion*. Routledge.

Loudon, I., Horder, J., & Webster, C. (1998). *General practice under the national health service 1948–1997*. Oxford University Press.

OED. (2023). s.v. "hermeneutic" (adj. & n.). In *Oxford English Dictionary* (p. 217). Oxford University Press.

Otto, W. (1979). *The homeric gods: The spiritual significance of Greek religion*. Thames and Hudson.

Pellauer, D., & Dauenhauer, B. (2022). *Paul Ricoeur*. Retrieved 24/07/2024 from https://plato.stanford.edu/entries/ricoeur/

Sackett, D., Rosenberg, W., Gray, J., Haynes, R., & Richardson, W. (1996). Evidence based medicine: What it is and what it isn't. *British Medical Journal, 312*, 71–72.

Shah, R., Clarke, R., Ahluwalia, S., & Launer, J. (2021). Finding meaning in the consultation: Working in the hermeneutic window. *British Journal of General Practice, 71*(707), 282–283.

Siegfried, T. (2017). *Philosophical critique exposes flaws in medical evidence hierarchies*. Retrieved 23/07/2024 from https://www.sciencenews.org/blog/context/critique-medical-evidence-hierarchies

Taylor, S. (1954). Good general practice. Oxford University Press.

Zimmermann, J. (2015). *Hermeneutics: A very short introduction*. Oxford University Press.

3   Nudging the status quo

Emma Ladds, Melissa Sayer and Rupal Shah

In this chapter, we consider how we can create meaning within the current context of healthcare, where measurable targets and outcomes are privileged and the drive to standardise is powerful. We will consider the tensions that arise when applying a hermeneutic frame within this paradigm and outline possible consequences and responses.

The famous business theorist, W. Edwards Deming (Hunter, 2015), is well known for his cynical reflection, 'A bad system will beat a good person every time.' At times, many of us might have found ourselves agreeing and feeling that there is no way to challenge the status quo. Not only do the actions of one individual often have a relatively small impact on the wider system, but even engaging in such a struggle can come at considerable personal cost. The experience of whistleblowers in the National Health Service (Hughes, 2023), the Royal Mail Scandal (Walker, 2024) and the outcome of the Infected Blood Inquiry (Reed, 2024) all speak to the challenges of taking on 'the system.'

And yet systems do not exist in isolation. The network of processes, activities and rules, the aims and values of the system are all determined by the interactions of those working within it. Culture is created by multiple such encounters (Spicer et al., 2021). Making sense of our place within this web of relationships and deriving meaning from our interactions can be a complex, challenging and frustrating endeavour. But we propose that not doing so carries the risk of moral injury and burn out.

Let us first consider examples of how the privileging of standardisation and measurement may affect individual clinicians and teams. Take John, a final-year medical student. He is over the moon to have just passed his final exams – it feels like a huge relief after six years of medical school, with an inexorable accumulation of debt. But now, he will finally start work as a doctor. He's looking forward to it, albeit with trepidation – he's waited a long time. But he doesn't know where he will be placed and has no control over this, which makes him anxious. Anxious about the team, the job, but most of all, where he is going to live. There are only a couple of months until he starts and before then, he has to relocate his entire life. What he hasn't yet internalised is that this is only the first move. For the next ten years or so, depending on the specialty he chooses, he will be moving every year. A house, community, stable family, these are things that will likely remain beyond his reach.

Now let us consider an idea recently put forward by a local Integrated Care Board (ICB). It was a good idea in principle. The ICB wanted to support all local

DOI: 10.4324/9781003517665-3

GP practices to have a training afternoon every three months. It offered to provide the necessary cover to enable practices to close for 'team training.' In return, the ICB proposed a remote training webinar that all staff would be expected to log onto. The webinar would outline the current activities and priorities of the ICB and help individuals understand local challenges and future directions of travel. The first training day went ahead, and the practices closed as planned. But not a single practice joined the remote webinar and the ICB presentation went unwatched.

So, what do John and the unwatched webinar have in common? Both are cases where 'the system' has tried to implement ideas that might work well for 'the system.' Of course, it is a good idea to have trainees who rotate – they will learn from different hospitals and teams, unpopular locations or specialties won't struggle to recruit a workforce and last-minute adjustments can be made for unexpected circumstances such as maternity or sickness leave. Efficiency can be maintained.

Similarly, of course, practice teams will benefit from understanding local strategic challenges and priorities – how else will they know where to direct their efforts to best support the system?

What such approaches overlook is that individuals derive meaning from system processes and interventions and ascribe meaning to their own interpretations (MacLeod et al., 2023). John feels as though he is simply a number and that he no longer matters as an individual. The system does not recognise that he has personal commitments and obligations. It does not recognise the stress of organising multiple moves. It ignores the fast pace of the local rental sector, the isolation of being relegated to a part of the country where he has no roots, the associated cost of the long train rides – both financial and emotional. Although we know that being part of a supportive team and having a sense of belonging improves metrics like postgraduate exam success (Roe et al., 2019), none of this has been factored in. John's interpretation is that he has no value. He is eminently replaceable. John resigns – a few months or years into his medical career.

It is a story replicated time and time again across the NHS in many different settings. A failure of policy makers to consider how individuals will ascribe meaning to the actions of 'the system.' In this case, such an approach contributes to the ever-increasing recruitment crisis, persistent strikes and low staff morale with which the health service is confronted, but there are many similar examples with equally impactful consequences.

What seems like a good idea to the ICB – a way of driving process efficiencies and priorities – again fails through a lack of hermeneutic appreciation. Not only has the ICB failed to consider what *meaningful training* might look like from a practice perspective, but it has also overlooked one of the most challenging aspects of hermeneutics – linguistics and the associated cultural associations. For example, for staff, 'team training day' conveys a sense of team bonding and learning. There's a 'day out' sense to the word, a 'school trip' vibe, an afternoon that should prove more enjoyable (or at least less stressful) than a standard afternoon of clinical practice. A 'strategic, local webinar' inherently conflicts with this implicit meaning. It conveys disconnection, remoteness, irrelevance – and ultimately results in a lack of attendance.

Endless examples abound, both within and beyond the NHS, of cases where prioritising the system's aims, i.e. to achieve its objectives in an efficient, cost-effective manner, overlooks the value a hermeneutic understanding can offer. Failure to consider such a fundamental part of being human, and in doing so, over-looking the essential observation that systems *are* interconnected individuals often results in costly inefficiencies and stress for leaders or policymakers.

Now, we will consider some clinician-patient encounters and describe how context impacts meaning. We will outline the inherent tensions between working within a bureaucratic, over-burdened system while also trying to give attention and care to individual patients.

Case 1   – The letter

This is an excerpt from a hypothetical 'e-consult' – a form-based, online consultation and triage platform, widely used in primary care in England, which requires patients to enter information about their problem before being given an appointment.

'*What do you need?*' A doctor's letter.
'*Please explain*' I need a letter saying I will need to miss days of university unpre-
    dictably due to my asthma and anxiety.'

As the on-call GP, should I accept this request at face value and write the let-ter? Send a brief paraphrase of the patient's sentence on signed, headed, electronic paper, as requested?
    Let me list the reasons to write this letter:

1   It would take me three minutes.
2   I am seven hours into a day which should be eight hours and 20 minutes long. Long ignored feelings in my abdomen remind me that I have not eaten or uri-nated. I still have 28 letters to read, action and code. Seventy-two prescriptions requests to respond to. There are nine emergency patients waiting, including a home visit request and a practice manager who needs support with a complaint. As usual, I predict that the day will be 13 hours long.
3   Saying 'no' may risk another complaint. Complaints take time to investigate and respond to, following due NHS process. More than three minutes.
4   Saying 'no' will mean creating time to speak to her, finding language to explore and explain. Energy to understand and collaborate. To plan. To care. The time and the emotional reserve.
5   Theoretically, as the letter is non-NHS work, our cash-strapped practice could charge for this letter, though we rarely do – a £20 income stream.
6   Most of my clinical decisions are made with patient autonomy in mind. The patient is an adult, with capacity to make decisions and she wants the letter.
7   Perhaps the generous response is to write the letter. Perhaps she would be helped by it, helped out of a tricky situation; maybe it will allow her to access more support from her university. She might feel she has an ally.

I look at her notes: no red flags. From what we know, her asthma and mental health appear 'not too bad.'

Alternatively, perhaps I might just reply to say no.

Perhaps, to quote a colleague, this request is 'Peak Gen Z'?

How might the university, her peers and her tutors be affected by sanctioned, unpredictable attendance?

Perhaps I could reply by text, signposting the asthma clinic and offering the link for self-referral to talking therapies for her anxiety. A packet of information sent. The patient is thereby 'informed,' 'supported' and 'educated' electronically. My role being to triage, to process her request, to signpost. Job done.

Or perhaps we might never know what's best. Perhaps I might never know her. This 19-year-old in London for the first time, trying to manage her university life.

What has happened that has led to her request? What might be underpinning her issues at university? What might she really need? How varied are her challenges and struggles? What does she need to know, to have, to be able to carry on? How much might we be able to make a difference as she navigates all this on her own? Would connection with a supportive health professional, a relationship with a trusted GP, be something that makes her path clearer, her hurdles less daunting?

The GMC mandates kindness (GMC, 2024): 'Doctors must be kind.' But what would it take for kindness to be possible in a system of e-consults and overwhelming workload?

Case 2 – Intractable hiccups

He's got hiccups. Abdominal pain. And probably Irritable Bowel Syndrome (IBS). Jonah is 31.

Some months ago, someone spoke to him on the phone and 'took a medical history.' The documentation is thorough and clear. Jonah has experienced 'no red flags': no symptoms that suggest a sinister diagnosis, such as bleeding or weight loss. Blood and stool tests were arranged. These were 'reassuringly normal' according to the text he was sent. And that was that. Safe, effective, defensible care.

'Reassuringly normal': Reassuring for whom? No one wants disease, but Jonah has been left without an explanation or understanding of his symptoms; with no roadmap to signal what to expect, or any possible solutions. The normal blood tests feel anything but reassuring to him.

He has looked at the IBS patient information leaflet he was sent, attached to the text. He's tried modifying his diet. And accepted that 'stress' plays a part.

His pain and fear continue. So, after some time and many crampy gut-wrenching days, he books another consultation.

What are you most concerned about? Another doctor asks, on the phone.

I just want it to go away.

Have you tried the FODMAPS diet (Bertin et al., 2024)? The buscopan? The link to access cognitive behavioural therapy?

Yes. Yes. Yes.

Does Citalopram help?

No.

And now some important questions. *Don't worry, we have to ask everyone these questions.*

**Are you suicidal?

**Would you like to discuss a crisis plan?

**Do you want to see the social prescriber?

Yes or No.

These important questions are double-asterisked within the computer-based depression review. This review must be completed because Jonah is on the practice's 'Depression Register' due to his Citalopram prescription. If double-asterisked questions and their corresponding tick boxes are not completed, the depression review does not count. Not counting means targets are missed and work done by the GP team is not paid.

In the past, in my practice, we often chose to ignore these tick boxes: we chose not to implement PHQ-9s (Kroenke et al., 2001) and GAD-7s (Spitzer et al., 2006) – tick box mood assessment questionnaires that sound like Star Wars characters. Quizzes that imply someone's despair and crisis can be measured and understood in less than two minutes, from their numerical responses to a Likert Scale. But nowadays not being paid risks not being viable: a practice that cannot remain open, cannot recruit new staff, cannot retain current staff. The targets must be met, the boxes must be ticked.

The pink box in the corner of the screen reminds the doctor of the necessary targets and work that needs to be done in the consultation. The depression review prompt disappears from the screen when the template is filled in. Job done.

Yet Jonah's pain and fear continue.

No clinician has been in the same room as him, built a connection, formed a relationship. No one has touched him, examined his abdomen, laid on hands. No one has expressed a wish to walk alongside him as this gets figured out, to help him bear it, to reassure him it is not his fault and it will get better.

Buried somewhere in the notes is free text stating that his brother was murdered three years ago. There is no clinical code for this, but still, the body keeps score (Van der Kolk, 2014). That's what someone might know, if they knew.

Kindness, gentleness, soothing, hope, warmth, kinship, allyship, space. None of these are tick boxes on the Depression Review. None are recognised or renumerated. But issuing a patient information leaflet about self-care during a depressive episode is.

Case 3   – Medication review overdue

It's a red font message at the bottom of the medication screen.

The responsible doctor has opened today's 72 repeat prescription requests. These are medications requested patients outside consultation time. Most list several medications, meaning that well over 100 decisions need to be made.

To prescribe, or not to prescribe?

Each of these decisions might be life-threatening for the patient. Or career-ending for the doctor, should dangerous errors be made. The responsibility for the medication lies with the issuing clinician.

With so many decisions to make every day, is there ever time to really 'review' the medication? Review it with the patient and make a shared, sensible, safe decision? How many hours per day would that take? What impact on waiting times and access to GP appointments would that have?

So instead, what are the doctor's likely responses to this red font prompt?

1   A text message 'please book a medication review' is sent to the patient.
2   The doctor clicks 'medication review done' having reviewed the notes.
3   The prompt gets ignored till next time.

What does a medication review mean?

It's a clinical discussion with the patient about their medication, reviewing their progress, giving information, exploring any side effects. Issues such as polypharmacy, interactions and over-prescribing may all be addressed in a proper medication review.

It sounds straightforward, particularly now that in the UK, many GP practices have pharmacists working within the practice team. But why do so many people take so many medications?

Guideline-driven healthcare, where it's difficult to have diabetes or survive a heart attack without at least four tablets forever, that's one reason. But why else might the prescriptions be mounting up? A billion items issued from primary care alone? (Mahase, 2021).

And from the clinician's side of the consulting room, why does it feel so hard to avoid prescribing? So hard to step down polypharmacy?

I pick up snippets from a helpful podcast discussion (Primary Care Knowledge Boost, 2024): follow a structured medication review checklist. Inform patients of risks, educate them about side effects. Get them 'on board.'

Is this true? Is information and 'education' what is lacking for the patient? And time what is lacking for the clinician? Would more education and more time equal less prescribing?

I also wonder what meaning medications have for doctors and their patients. Might considering hermeneutics help? I think of patients I know. I ask some of them. I speak to other doctors and to pharmacists.

For the patient, perhaps the tablets mean:

1   Something can be done to help me, which will make me live longer.
2   I am being cared for.
3   I can go to my doctor and pharmacist for check-ups.
4   My illness is genuine and people believe me.
5   Side effects are to be expected but are almost comforting, like a pharmaceutical hug. Like a numbing.

6 I won't be told, 'Your condition is not bad enough to require medication, so we reject your application for benefits.'

For the doctor, perhaps the tablets mean:

1 I know what to do in this situation.
2 I can help this person, there is something I can offer, there is hope.
3 The patient can see I am taking their suffering seriously.
4 The end of the consultation is signalled, like a party bag.
5 I need not engage with this suffering. Medication is easier and quicker to issue than time and emotional labour.

Imagine a patient you care about, who has chronic back pain saying, 'I am literally begging you for codeine so I can function.' Or, 'the only thing that helps me is the Pregabalin.'

Their medication page looks like this (Figure 3.1):

Is it straightforward for a doctor to decline these requests? Guidelines tell us we should (NICE, 2021). But the guideline is not witnessing this suffering and distress. It is not respecting this adult who knows what they need. It is not experiencing the feelings of helplessness in the room.

Might one hope to try an alternative approach? Informed by making meaning?

An acknowledgement of the immense pain suffered by the patient and an exploration of its impact and associated fears. A willingness to continue to explore, validate and address the suffering. Curiosity and care. Reassurance given by explanations of what is (and is not) happening inside the body when it hurts. A declaration of wanting to help, to do the best for someone, to ensure they are safe and cared for, heard and supported. Hopefully empowered and engaged. Both parties accepting the limitations of what can be safely offered on prescription?

Is this possible in the time allowed, with the energy the clinician has in their demanding day? And if it is not, how much more time might it cost in the long

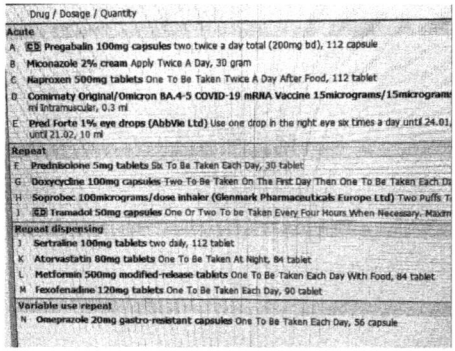

Drug / Dosage / Quantity
Acute
A **Pregabalin** 100mg capsules two twice a day total (200mg bd), 112 capsule
B Miconazole 2% cream Apply Twice A Day, 30 gram
C Naproxen 500mg tablets One To Be Taken Twice A Day After Food, 112 tablet
D Comirnaty Original/Omicron BA.4-5 COVID-19 mRNA Vaccine 15micrograms/15micrograms ml Intramuscular, 0.3 ml
E Pred Forte 1% eye drops (AbbVie Ltd) Use one drop in the right eye six times a day until 24.01, until 21.02, 10 ml
Repeat
F Prednisolone 5mg tablets Six To Be Taken Each Day, 30 tablet
G Doxycycline 100mg capsules Two To Be Taken On The First Day Then One To Be Taken Each Da
H Soprobec 100micrograms/dose inhaler (Glenmark Pharmaceuticals Europe Ltd) Two Puffs T
J Tramadol 50mg capsules One Or Two To Be Taken Every Four Hours When Necessary. Maxim
Repeat dispensing
J Sertraline 100mg tablets two daily, 112 tablet
K Atorvastatin 80mg tablets One To Be Taken At Night, 84 tablet
L Metformin 500mg modified-release tablets One To Be Taken Each Day With Food, 84 tablet
M Fexofenadine 120mg tablets One To Be Taken Each Day, 90 tablet
Variable use repeat
N Omeprazole 20mg gastro-resistant capsules One To Be Taken Each Day, 56 capsule

Figure 3.1 Medication Screen on Computerised Medical Record (Sayer, 2024; Photo).

term, in consultation time and monitoring? How many more prescriptions issued? How much more risk taken, for both patient and doctor and for the planet?

A Mother's perspective

Our 20-year-old son, who is training to be a personal trainer, works in a gym, is physically extremely fit, and is the son of two doctors, presented with a ten-day history of dizziness and feeling lightheaded. In A&E, he was found to have a severe iron deficiency anaemia (haemoglobin of 82g/L), requiring admission to hospital for an iron infusion. Having collapsed in A&E he was told he had 'won himself an endoscopy as an inpatient,' so he stayed overnight, having had his infusion. He was then sent home and told to wait for further appointments. He was unsure whether he could return to work.

Within the first month of being home he had a colonoscopy, which was normal. He then heard nothing further from either primary or secondary care. We submitted an e-consultation request to the (otherwise excellent) GP surgery, one from my son, and a separate one from me, both requesting a GP face-to-face follow up appointment for support and care and some help in navigating next steps. On separate days, we both received text messages from different triage GPs stating that 'it was all in hand in gastroenterology in secondary care.' In neither response was our son offered either a call or a face-to-face appointment. I waited a further two weeks and then, reluctantly, sent an email to the gastroenterology consultant to expedite next steps. This has resulted in two further investigations and one pending.

Three months since his admission, there has been no offer of a face-to-face appointment. My son remains none the wiser about the cause of the symptoms, and no one has spoken to him or examined him. He has been offered no guidance or support from general practice and no nutritional or dietetic input.

While I remain concerned about the well-being of our son, two points have struck me about the state of our current NHS systems.

First, where is the curiosity of the doctors investigating him? Even given the limitations and pressures of the NHS, no one seems to feel that exploring what has made a 20 year old so unwell is important. What happens to inspired, intelligent and caring medical students to reduce them to disinterested and apparently uninquisitive and uncaring doctors?

Second, where is the care for my son? The lack of face-to-face contact, both in primary and secondary care, has a significant impact. It is invalidating. The underlying message to my son is that his illness is of no concern, and he is of no value.

At a stage in life where he should be flourishing and learning to fly, he is held back in a system where no doctor is holding his hand, reassuring him, being his advocate, being curious on his behalf, understanding the context of his life, or teaching him that he matters.

Lucy Andrews, GP in South London

Conclusion

Era 2 medicine (Berwick, 2016) requires the generation of data, regulation and adherence to guidelines. An inadvertent consequence is remoteness, disconnection and alienation. Perhaps partly because of this, access has become politicised – yet focusing only the time taken to respond rather the quality of the response is misleading. As clinicians, we have a choice about how to respond to individual patients and to our colleagues. Healthcare policy can and should be written to encourage more thoughtful practice. This may mean allowing longer appointments, seeing fewer patients and allowing time for staff to come together to discuss some of the moral dilemmas they face – as highlighted in the cases above. This approach may result in short term loss but is likely to lead in the longer term to more sustainable, personalised care provision. Perhaps we should attempt to escape from the 'scarcity loop' (Shah & Launer, 2019), a way of thinking that encourages us to use 'enough' or 'not enough' as the measure by which we judge how to allocate all resource – including love, time, care and attention. A hermeneutic approach challenges this paradigm and the notion that rationing our humanity leads to more efficient healthcare systems. In the cases discussed in this chapter, a hermeneutic approach might involve:

- Considering a de-centralised approach to junior doctor training that encourages doctors to work in an area they understand and which they consider to be 'home'; with proportional recruitment from deprived areas.
- Rethinking the value of 'mandatory training' and only retaining training which is supported by staff feedback as producing helpful new understanding or changing practice.
- Promoting staff training that considers the moral dilemmas that we are faced with on a daily basis and that encourages conversations about how to respond in a way that is congruent with team values.
- Incentivising meaningful clinician-patient relationships, for example with use of questionnaires such as the 'Care Measure' (Mercer et al., 2005).
- Incentivising Healthcare Institutions to retain and value their staff.
- Considering how and when remote consultations save time and resources and conversely, when personal contact is likely to be kinder and more effective.

References

Bertin, L., Zanconato, M., Crepaldi, M., Marasco, G., Cremon, C., Barbara, G., Barberio, B., Zingone, F., & Savarino, E. (2024). The role of the FODMAP diet in IBS. *Nutrients*, *16*(3), 370.

Berwick, D. (2016). Era 3 for medicine and health care. *Journal of the American Medical Association*, *315*(13), 1329–1330.

GMC. (2024). *Good medical practice*. Retrieved 13/06/2024 from https://www.gmc-uk.org/professional-standards/good-medical-practice-2024

Hughes, D. (2023). *NHS whistleblowers need more protection, expert warns*. Retrieved 09/06/2024 from https://www.bbc.co.uk/news/health-66051884

Hunter, J. (2015). *A bad system will beat a good person every time.* Retrieved 09/06/2024 from https://deming.org/a-bad-system-will-beat-a-good-person-every-time/

Kroenke, K., Spitzer, R. L., & Williams, J. B. (2001). The PHQ-9: Validity of a brief depression severity measure. *Journal of General Internal Medicine, 16*(9), 606–613.

MacLeod, M., McCaffrey, G., Wilson, E., Zimmer, L., Snadden, D., Zimmer, P., Jónatansdóttir, S., Fyfe, T, Koopmans, E., & Ulrich, C. (2023). Exploring the intersection of hermeneutics and implementation: A scoping review. *Systematic Reviews, 12*(1), 30.

Mahase, E. (2021). Overprescribing: 10% of items dispensed in primary care are inappropriate, review finds. *BMJ, 374*(2338). https://doi.org/10.1136/bmj.n2338

Mercer, S., McConnachie, A., Maxwell, M., Heaney, D., & Watt, G. (2005). Relevance and practical use of the Consultation and Relational Empathy (CARE) Measure in general practice. *Family Practice, 22*(3), 328–334.

NICE. (2021). *Chronic pain (primary and secondary) in over 16s: Assessment of all chronic pain and management of chronic primary pain.* Retrieved 09/06/2024 from https://www.nice.org.uk/guidance/ng193

Primary Care Knowledge Boost. (2024). Polypharmacy. In *Primary care knowledge boost.* https://pckb.org/e/polypharmacy/

Reed, J. (2024). *What is the infected blood scandal and will victims get compensation?* Retrieved 09/06/2024 from https://www.bbc.co.uk/news/health-48596605

Roe, V., Patterson, F., Kerrin, M., & Edwards, H. (2019). *What supported your success in training? A qualitative exploration of the factors associated with an absence of an ethnic attainment gap in post-graduate specialty training.* General Medical Council.

Sayer, M. (2024). *Medication screen on computerised medical record* (photo).

Shah, R., & Launer, J. (2019). Escaping the scarcity loop. *The Lancet, 394*(10193), 112–113.

Spicer, J., Ahluwalia, S., & Shah, R. (2021). Moral flux in primary care: The effect of complexity. *Journal of Medical Ethics, 47*(2), 86–89.

Spitzer, R., Kroenke, K., Williams, J., & Löwe, B. (2006). A brief measure for assessing generalized anxiety disorder: The GAD-7. *Archives of Internal Medicine, 166*(10), 1092–1097.

Van der Kolk, B. (2014). *The body keeps the score: Brain, mind, and body in the healing of trauma.* Penguin Books.

Walker, P. (2024). *What is the UK's Post Office IT scandal about and who is involved?* Retrieved 09/06/2024 from https://www.theguardian.com/uk-news/2024/jan/11/what-is-uk-post-office-horizon-it-scandal-about-who-involved

4 Hermeneutic approaches in complex multimorbidity

Sophie Park and Martina Ann Kelly

Hermeneutic approaches in complex multimorbidity

Increasing numbers of people are living with multiple illnesses, but their care is often fragmented (Smith et al., 2012). Both our healthcare systems and ways of clinically educating clinicians tend to focus on 'one problem at a time.' In contrast, patients are often juggling several priorities. They experience the burden of their illnesses, but also the burden of treatment, balancing multiple medications, hospital services and healthcare providers, while attending to their daily lives and basic self-care – exercise, diet, rest, family life, striving for 'work-life-balance' (Ørtenblad et al., 2018). Harmonising personal circumstances, priorities and preferences requires thoughtful attention and an active intention to adapt care to an individual's particular situation.

Generalists are well placed to support people living with undifferentiated and multiple illnesses, to provide person-centred attention and co-ordination of care (Barnett et al., 2012; Muth et al., 2019; Salisbury et al., 2018). However, the '*how to*' of what that looks like in the '*swampy lowlands*' (Schon) of clinical praxis and how to support learning to maximise adaptable and personalised care remains a challenge (Bansal et al., 2022). In this chapter, we explore hermeneutics as an interpretive approach that can support patients, physicians and the multiprofessional team as they navigate the complex demands of living with multiple illnesses. To demonstrate the craft of hermeneutic engagement, which involves key concepts such as the willingness to understand and engage in dialogue, we draw on our experience as general practitioners, as we consider the care of Gisella, and introduce a metaphor of weaving, drawing parallels between weaving cloth and the back-and-forth dialogue between patient and healthcare team that co-constructs a unique, context and person-specific fabric of illness, and health experience, over time.

Weaving hermeneutic possibilities

Gadamer, a German philosopher introduced in Chapter 1, advocated hermeneutics as an approach to help society navigate the challenges of living in a complex world. In his text Enigma of Health (Gadamer, 1996), he suggests that health is experienced as a state of harmony, of being in the world, manifested 'precisely by virtue

DOI: 10.4324/9781003517665-4

of escaping our attention' (p. 96). Illness can disturb our sense of well-being and capacity to be actively engaged in the world; shifting the 'harmonious interplay between the feeling of well-being and our capacity to be actively engaged in the world' (p. 99). The hermeneutic task of the physician and healthcare team is to work with the patient to restore a sense of equilibrium. This requires a skilled hand and a 'sensitive ear which is attentive to the significance of what the patient says' (p. 99). This intentional praxis recognises that the patient is already self-interpreting and embedded in a world of relational meanings. Conversation with others, such as clinicians, can help to realise a new or re-framed understanding of their experiences (Aho, 2021, pp. 177–187).

To apply some key concepts from Gadamerian hermeneutics, we use the metaphor of weaving, interlacing vertical strands of person, place and problem (the warp) woven with the back-and-forth movement of generalist-hermeneutic principles of care (the weft). See Figure 4.1.

Using this metaphor, we illustrate how physician and patient co-construct patterns together as an inductive, responsive process that evolves over time. Weaving becomes a way to recognise wholeness in health by overcoming seemingly broken connections, to create tapestries of shared meaning and well-being. While an industrialised approach might prioritise identical, standardised multiple garments, a weaver's aim is to produce artefacts which vary in character and purpose, to meet the particular needs of a person at that place and time. Some of the materials (e.g. thread) used by the weaver might use industrial-produced resources, but the application of these within a garment requires technical skill, creativity and mastery of knowledge about the process and their client (Kneebone, 2020). This balance of repeatable, standardised production, with the agility and creativity to produce something unique (and beautiful) for a particular purpose and person, is complex. There is no one right or perfect garment. Rather, an artefact is appreciated in relation to its feasibility (e.g. cost) and value as being fit for purpose: be that aesthetic, functional or both. This weaving requires experience, skill and knowledge relevant to the weaver's own

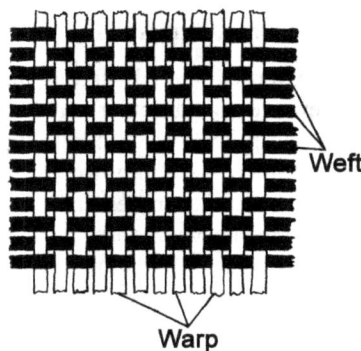

Figure 4.1 Warp and Weft in Weaving (Foresman, 2019).

professional expertise, but also an ability to connect and align with the broader needs of an individual, community or society.

Weaving with Gisella: Gisella's lifeworld

Gisella, aged 38, attends her GP surgery for a medication review. She has rheumatoid arthritis (RA), hypothyroidism, eczema, asthma, polycystic ovarian syndrome and anxiety. She is married, with a seven-year-old daughter, Sara, who also has asthma. She has been trying for some time to get pregnant. She works as an administrator and her husband is a construction worker. Since her diagnosis of RA three years ago, Gisella has experienced several flares of her RA; recurrent pain in her ankles, shoulders and hands make mornings particularly difficult as she struggles to get her daughter ready for school and to get into work. She is presently on an immunosuppressant, which is meant to slow her disease progression. She was very concerned about the side effects of starting this, but after several relapses and courses of steroids, felt she had no choice but to take it. She continues to worry about possible side effects, and if it will impact her ability to have more children. She wonders why her body is attacking itself. Being unwell has resulted in prolonged periods of time out of work, and her employer is not very understanding – it is hard for her to get time off for her monitoring blood tests and different healthcare appointments. She is worried about the mortgage – it felt well within reach when the couple bought their flat, but with her being intermittently out of work, finances are tight. She isn't sleeping well. She wonders if she should change her anti-anxiety medication and has been using some of her mother's 'relaxing pills' which she finds very effective. She has brought along several studies which show benefits of use of complementary medicine and asks your opinion.

The warp: this person, in this place, in this time

In weaving, the warp refers to vertical threads. In our analogy, the warp is represented by Gisella and her lifeworld – a particular person, in a particular place and time, with specific concerns and problems. Gisella is juggling not only a list of illnesses, but how they impact upon her ability to live the life she wants. While Gisella is benefitting from her immunosuppressant, she is concerned about the long-term sequalae. She has skipped several doses and started some vitamins recommended by a naturopath. Yet, she is unsure how safe the vitamins are and wants to be able to understand all these different treatments and their potential interplay. She wonders if she should discuss her worries about her ability to manage work and her financial worries with her doctor – will the doctor be interested? And how can they help, anyway? Most of all, she really wants another baby. Time is ticking by, and it has always been her dream to have a family. Within these tensions, we can grasp how good clinical care is not just through the logarithmic application of 'facts,' flowsheets, guidelines and outcome measurements, but instead through establishing their relevance to deeply intertwined human ideas, concerns, and expectations. While patient-centred practice and communication skills training has done much to advance the importance of soliciting and acknowledging these fundamental aspects of Gisella's lifeworld (Brown et al., 1986; Kurtz et al., 2005), it has sometimes fallen short of providing tools for how to *integrate* these insights within clinical care. This is what the hermeneutic window opens (Shah et al., 2020; Figure 4.2); how patients and healthcare providers can work together to find and co-create meaning, even in the face of what seem irresolvable conflicts.

This process requires curiosity and courage. A common response to something unfamiliar is to draw back and establish difference or otherness, protecting our own legitimacy or institutional belonging. Arthur Frank talks about clinicians behaving as 'artificial persons,' who represent their institution rather than themselves, by using bureaucratic language and adopting generic approaches to patients (Frank, 2005).

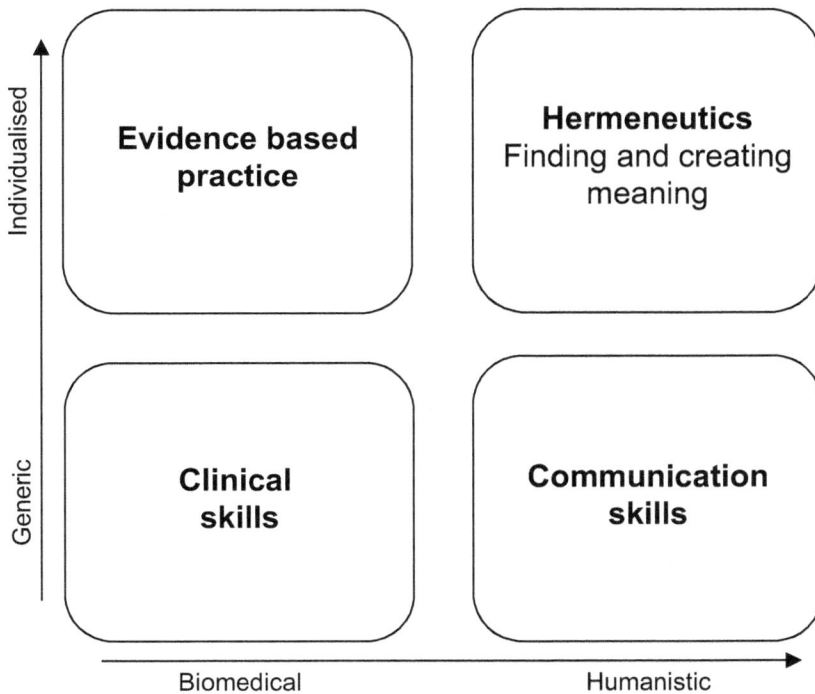

Figure 4.2 The Four Domain Model (Shah et al., 2020).

Instead, hermeneutics requires us to lean in and explore, exchange and share commonalities. We have to let go of our familiar way of interpreting the world, as being the 'right' way, and see it as conditional, as one of many possibilities (Park & Leedham-Green, 2024). This enables us to appreciate, respect and connect with other, perhaps contrasting ways of making meaning, and understand how these frame experiences, values and knowledge differently. Experiential knowledge of the patient or practitioner might therefore shift from being 'less important' than medicine adherence, and instead become an enmeshed, complex interplay to explore and engage.

The weft: hermeneutic principles of care

Now, we weave ideas of Gadamerian hermeneutics horizontally, moving back and forth to illustrate how generalist hermeneutic approaches to praxis offer possibilities for Gisella's care.

From the way Gisella is sitting, very upright and tense, her rapid speech, it is apparent to the clinician that a simple re-issuing of a prescription is not the topic of this consultation, nor the most appropriate approach to help Gisella, despite the stated reason for the appointment. A key skill of hermeneutic practice is to notice and respond to these cues. The physician needs to engage with and better understand how she is thinking and what is going on in her life.

Her physician takes a breath, centres herself with a brief pause, and invites –

'How are things?', 'tell me more'

A willingness to understand

Understanding, in the first instance, requires a willingness to understand; that is a sensibility to being open, to being wrong and to revising and re-interpreting the topic under discussion. This demands a curiosity to seek beyond the immediately apparent, to 'inductively forage', that is, where patients are invited to freely unfold their reason for the encounter and the physician then follows the patient's lead (Donner-Banzhoff et al., 2017; Michiels-Corsten et al., 2022). In this way, 'routine' questions of 'history-taking' are dynamically co-constructed and evolve with the patient. The pattern is unknown, the moment-to-moment interaction determining what will emerge. This exchange requires attention not only to the present moment, but also the patient's context, community, culture, historical roots and future aspirations. Similarly, the clinician requires a critical awareness of how their professional and personal experiences shape their approach, and humility to draw upon their networks and team expertise.

Dialogue

The physician probes further

Can you help me understand what this feels like, and what it means for you? (Aho, 2021)

To explore all of Gisella's ideas, concerns and expectations is likely beyond the scope of a time-pressed clinician in a single visit. However, the possibilities to understand are extended by continuity (offering follow up) and working in a team-setting. As the team work with the many dimensions of Gisella's issues, care becomes shared, to involve multiple perspectives and foci of knowledge, as a distributed hermeneutics.

Hermeneutic approaches to clinician-patient interactions acknowledge the possibility of multiple understandings and interpretations of an issue. Applying hermeneutic principles to caring for patients with multiple illnesses, reframes the 'consultation' as a 'conversation.' That is, an exchange where two people engage with the topic under discussion, as a subject of importance to them (the health of the patient). The goal is not didactic transfer about persuading or convincing somebody, by expounding a (medical) point of view, rather it is about pursing the conditional truth of the matter together. How is she, what's going on, in this moment at this time. 'Dialogue and discussion,' as Gadamer writes, 'serve to humanize the fundamentally unequal relationship that prevails between doctor and patient' (Gadamer, 1996). Dialogue means 'through words,' an interchange between two people, which contrasts with the dominance of a culture of monologue, where 'doctor knows best' – where we listen but do not hear each other.

Gadamer uses the term 'play' to demonstrate how, when 'in play,' players become preoccupied with the game (or topic) or creative exchange, rather than with who wins (Gadamer, 2013). Gisella's health becomes something important to both her and her physician. Curiosity delves into what it 'is' to live with multiple illnesses. To perceive Gisella's lifeworld as multi-dimensional, beyond social categorisation of 'woman,' 'mother,' 'wife,' 'daughter,' 'administrator,' 'patient,' 'middle-class,' 'married,' 'sick,' 'having chronic illness,' 'having auto-immune diseases,' 'stressed' to view all such experiences as 'in relation to' her unique context and all its nuances and complexities – this person, in this place, with this problem(s). This is 'hermeneutic realism,' where Gisella's world is pregnant with meaning, more that we can ever say or know. The idea of dialogue is not to pin meaning down but to *expand and develop possibilities* of what they *may* mean by giving life to new insights as Gisella, her physician and healthcare team work together over time. In this way, understanding is never finite; there is never a 'single' best answer, but many possibilities to understand.

Gisella's care becomes more comprehensive. The pharmacist works to explore Gisella's concerns about her medication after a conversation with the GP who first saw her. The social prescriber advises her on benefits and financial supports, also providing some supportive counselling. The first point of contact physiotherapist provides tips on managing stiffness and pain. Gisella is eligible for an exercise and mobility programme for people with chronic diseases at her local gym, which can provide child-care while she attends it. The GP emails Gisella's rheumatologist and asks about the implications of taking the immunosuppressant on future pregnancies and relays his response to Gisella. She also advises Gisella about reviewing her dose of thyroxine if she does become pregnant.

Horizons of understanding

Working hermeneutically is about expanding understanding. Each time we gain a new perspective, we re-evaluate our prior conceptions, enhancing our understanding, seeing familiar things in new ways. As Gisella and her healthcare team work together, both benefit. Co-construction is about exchange – her physician and healthcare team gain a new perspective, as they develop more expanded views of illness and what health and suffering are; and what the possibilities are of 'being with' a patient instead of simply trying to 'fix' them.

Land and Meyer highlight the importance of transformatory learning: how the way in which we understand or 'see' something can change. Both clinician and patient are open to learning and adapting each other's knowledge, to formulate a problem and potential solutions in new ways. This might prove challenging for one/other or both, and both might occupy a 'liminal' space for a period of time, where they dip into new ways of seeing or understanding, but revert to more familiar territory. Over time, however, they grow the capacity and confidence to understand and formulate problems in new and creative ways. Transformational learning opportunities and possibilities are open to both clinician and patient, re-shaping meaning making through collective interactions with each other and beyond.

Hermeneutics is always 'on the way'

A year has passed. Gisella has an appointment to ask for a sick note. Her doctor, knowing the back story, is prepared to write one. But a first glance indicates that all is not as it seems. Gisella looks tired, pale and has lost weight.

The doctor looks at Gisella and asks, '*What's wrong?*'

Gisella responds, 'I had a miscarriage last week.' She breaks down and sobs. 'We were so happy when I finally got pregnant, and then this happens. I don't know if we'll get another chance.'

The doctor reaches over and puts her hand over Gisella's. They look at one another and it is clear to Gisella that the significance of what she has said has been understood. This implicit connection allows the doctor to move into asking some clinical questions. It transpires that Gisella didn't go to hospital when the bleeding started and hasn't told work what happened. The doctor is worried about the amount of blood Gisella has lost, but the bleeding has stopped now and her pulse and BP are normal, so an urgent blood test is arranged at the practice. Gisella stopped taking her immunosuppressant when she got pregnant and the doctor says she will liaise with Gisella's rheumatology specialist nurse.

They talk about the impact on Gisella's mood and when she might start trying again to conceive. Gisella gets a sick note, but at her request, 'miscarriage' is not entered as the cause for missing work. A follow up appointment is arranged and Gisella is aware that she should check her NHS app for the blood result the following day and that there is a chance she will need to go to hospital.

The task of hermeneutics is never done. As one challenge is overcome, a new one is presented. As new issues are revealed, old issues fade into the past, leaving a trace that may require fresh examination. Working hermeneutically is an investment and reward that ebbs and flows over time. There is no 'end' but only the possibility of an ongoing conversation. Gisella, her physician and healthcare team continue to work together, where the threads of the warp are woven intricately through the back-and-forth movements of hermeneutic weft, creating imaginative, richer and more complex patterns, a fabric that is never finished. The time, pace and tempo might vary, as might the person leading, following or fore-fronting an exchange, but patient and clinician can build upon and use their shared understandings together. These exchanges are not isolated, but part of a much wider and distributed web of interactions and learning, each bringing new experiences and insights to every encounter.

Conclusion

As knowledge evolves and we learn new ways to process and exchange this knowledge, so too will the possibilities for distributed hermeneutics develop. This is not inevitable, nor straightforward. As the world becomes more interconnected and our networks widen, we need to strengthen and utilise our critical awareness to inform each interaction with our patients. How do our thoughts, feelings and experiences shape our exchanges with others and what is the interplay (integration, dissonance, priorities, etc.) between different forms and types of knowledge? Currently, our focus has been almost exclusively upon the interplay of diseases (Álvarez-Gálvez et al., 2023; Head et al., 2021; NIHR Evidence, 2021; Pearson-Stuttard et al., 2019). However, as our understanding grows of the interconnections between physical, social and psychological experiences, we begin to see, for example, how physiological ageing is a product not just of time, but stress, social disadvantage and inequalities. Therefore, managing 'multiple conditions' might not just mean managing multiple diseases, but also multiple social determinants of health. 'Health' means something different to us all and exploring what health means to an individual at a particular time is a crucial element of distributed hermeneutics to support and challenge expectations. Learning how and when to adapt the knowledge and care we use, is as important as the knowledge and care itself. This dynamic and evolving approach to clinical practice is both challenging and exciting. How will your textile evolve, and how will it interweave, pass by or grow with other wider tapestries of life?

References

Aho, K. (2021). Gadamer and health. In T. D. George & G. J. van der Heiden (Eds.), *The Gadamerian mind* (pp. 177–187). Routledge.

Álvarez-Gálvez, J., Ortega-Martín, E., Carretero-Bravo, J., Pérez-Muñoz, C., Suárez-Lledó, V., & Ramos-Fiol, B. (2023). Social determinants of multimorbidity patterns: A systematic review. *Frontiers in Public Health, 11*, 1081518.

Bansal, A., Greenley, S., Mitchell, C., Park, S., Shearn, K., & Reeve, J. (2022). Optimising planned medical education strategies to develop learners' Person-Centredness: A realist review. *Medical Education, 56*(5), 489–503.

Barnett, K., Mercer, S. W., Norbury, M., Watt, G., Wyke, S., & Guthrie, B. (2012). Epidemiology of multimorbidity and implications for health care, research, and medical education: A cross-sectional study. *The Lancet, 380*(9836), 37–43.

Brown, J., Stewart, M., McCracken, E., McWhinney, I., & Levenstein, J. (1986). The patient-centred clinical method. 2. Definition and application. *Family Practice, 3*(2), 75–79.

Donner-Banzhoff, N., Seidel, J., Sikeler, A., Bösner, S., Vogelmeier, M., Westram, A., Feufel, M., Gaissmaier, W., Wegwarth, O., & Gigerenzer, G. (2017). The phenomenology of the diagnostic process: A primary care-based survey. *Medical Decision Making, 37*(1), 27–34.

Foresman, P. S. (2019). *Warp and weft (PSF)* (Diagram). Wikimedia Commons. Labels simplified by book editors. https://commons.wikimedia.org/wiki/File:Warp_and_weft

Frank, A. W. (2005). *The renewal of generosity: Illness, medicine, and how to live.* University of Chicago Press.

Gadamer, H.- G. (1996). *The enigma of health: The art of healing in a scientific age.* John Wiley & Sons.

Gadamer, H.- G. (2013). *Truth and method* (J. M. Weinsheimer & D. G. Marshall, Trans.). Bloomsbury Academic.

Head, A., Fleming, K., Kypridemos, C., Schofield, P., Pearson-Stuttard, J., & O'Flaherty, M. (2021). Inequalities in incident and prevalent multimorbidity in England, 2004–19: A population-based, descriptive study. *The Lancet Healthy Longevity, 2*(8), e489–e497. https://doi.org/10.1016/S2666-7568(21)00146-X

Kneebone, R. (2020). *Expert: Understanding the path to mastery.* Penguin UK.

Kurtz, S., Draper, J., & Silverman, J. (2005). *Teaching and learning communication skills in medicine.* CRC press.

Michiels-Corsten, M., Weyand, A., Gold, J., Bösner, S., & Donner-Banzhoff, N. (2022). Inductive foraging: Patients taking the lead in diagnosis, a mixed-methods study. *Family Practice*, *39*(3), 479–485.

Muth, C., Blom, J., Smith, S., Johnell, K., Gonzalez-Gonzalez, A., Nguyen, T., Brueckle, M., Cesari, M., Tinetti, M., & Valderas, J. (2019). Evidence supporting the best clinical management of patients with multimorbidity and polypharmacy: A systematic guideline review and expert consensus. *Journal of Internal Medicine*, *285*(3), 272–288. https://doi.org/10.1111/joim.12842

NIHR Evidence. (2021). *Multiple long-term conditions (multimorbidity): Making sense of the evidence*. https://evidence.nihr.ac.uk/collection/making-sense-of-the-evidence-multiple-long-term-conditions-multimorbidity/

Ørtenblad, L., Meillier, L., & Jønsson, A. (2018). Multi-morbidity: A patient perspective on navigating the health care system and everyday life. *Chronic Illness*, *14*(4), 271–282.

Park, S., & Leedham-Green, K. (2024). *Generalism in clinical practice and education*. UCL Press. https://doi.org/https://doi.org/10.14324/111.9781800085428

Pearson-Stuttard, J., Ezzati, M., & Gregg, E. (2019). Multimorbidity—A defining challenge for health systems. *The Lancet Public Health*, *4*(12), e599–e600.

Salisbury, C., Man, M.-S., Bower, P., Guthrie, B., Chaplin, K., Gaunt, D. M., Brookes, S., Fitzpatrick, B., Gardner, C., & Hollinghurst, S. (2018). Management of multimorbidity using a patient-centred care model: A pragmatic cluster-randomised trial of the 3D approach. *The Lancet*, *392*(10141), 41–50.

Shah, R., Clarke, R., Ahluwalia, S., & Launer, J. (2020). Finding meaning in the consultation: Introducing the hermeneutic window. *British Journal of General Practice*, *70*(699), 502–503.

Smith, S., Soubhi, H., Fortin, M., Hudon, C., & O'Dowd, T. (2012). Managing patients with multimorbidity: Systematic review of interventions in primary care and community settings. *British Medical Journal*, *345*. https://doi.org/10.1136/bmj.e5205

5 Hermeneutic approaches in mental health and chronic pain

Jens Foell and Sami Timimi

Complex holding work

Consulting with patients who live with chronic pain is never just one thing – primary care work includes cognitive, administrative, organisational and emotional labour. The box of tissues to soak up tears belongs on a doctor's desk just as much as does a stethoscope, thermometer and pulse oximeter (Figure 5.1).

People in pain have long medication lists. Pain is rarely an isolated phenomenon, it comes as a package deal, with other mental, emotional, and social manifestations of distress. Letters must be written, medications managed, blood tests ordered. Administrative tasks are part of the maintenance aspect of 'holding work' (Cocksedge et al., 2011). Just as a housewife in premodern times maintained the house in functioning order, a huge amount of invisible, background work goes into keeping General Practice viable (Barnard et al., 2024).

GPs differ in whether they feel that General Practice is the right holding environment for the complexity that goes alongside chronic pain – often, there is

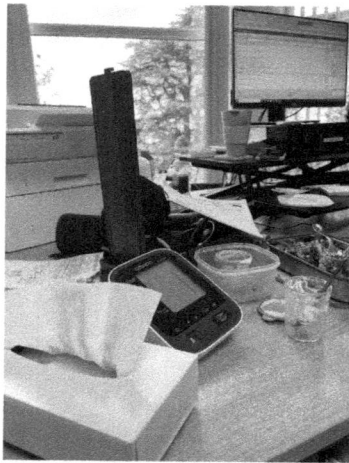

Figure 5.1 Still GP Life, Lunchtime at Work (Foell, 2024).

DOI: 10.4324/9781003517665-5

co-existing trauma and suffering. Some think these patients would be better off in a pain clinic or in an outpatient mental health clinic, where there is a clear epistemic framework and longer appointment times. The jury is out as to whether GPs are conveyors or containers, gatekeepers for secondary care or advocates for the patient. Regardless, they are certainly street-level bureaucrats with a regulated and governed discretionary space in which to make decisions (Lipsky, 1980).

The dilemma of how far a hermeneutic approach fits with street-level bureaucracy is discussed in the case studies below. Within a context that requires negotiation of the mundane alongside consideration of the existential, we refrain from romanticising the hermeneutic window as an entry point for a permanently changed relationship. We show that working within it can catalyse change, help stuck situations, or at least humanise them and therefore may prevent the clinician from resorting to potentially harmful interventions.

Debbie and Wendy – case studies illustrating 'stuckness'

Debbie was on my list again. I am familiar with Debbie's predicaments, including her chronic, all-over-body pain. Her sister was murdered. She then raised the children. Issues associated with this situation include referrals to Child and Adolescent Psychiatry for the bereaved children (which unfortunately always bounced back, rejected), bodily issues like high blood pressure, weight gain, plus the referrals, blood tests, etc., associated with having a long-term condition. On several occasions we had high stake-high-drama-encounters about the unbearableness of Debbie's fate. I remember these episodes of 'heavy emotional lifting' (C. Stannard, personal communication, 2022).

'This is killing me' is a common curtain-raiser. Unfortunately though, this is not about death, this is about torture, this is about staying alive in suffering. These consultations are like encounters in which the doctor is involved in torture, and their job is to ensure the torturers are not overdoing it. Sufferers plea for an escape from experiencing torture. This escape is envisaged as taking medication, as a referral to a situation that promises restitution or transformation, or as a simple respite, a city-break from being stuck in pain.

'Chronic pain' is a misleading term, perhaps coined by people who do not themselves live with pain. 'Chronic' implies that every day is the same, that pain is a stable and steady state. It suggests that clinicians should attempt to mitigate or erase or even fix the unbearableness of being in this state (Atkin, 2023).

Acceptance is the goal of most pain management programmes, which are offered as one-off-interventions. Acceptance is envisaged as a single event, like getting married, not as a fluctuating process. Over my many years of practice, I have concluded that there is no such thing as acceptance. My relationship with people in pain is longer than the outcome data from trials in pain management or analgesia. I observe more often a disordered amalgamation of the cycles of grief, where the different stages fail to arise in a logical, sequential order.

Debbie is back. We have been here before. She can't bear being here. She is fed up. If torture is about breaking people's sense of coherence she is at breaking point. She can't stand it anymore. She addresses me as the conduit for an escape. A re-referral? Changes in medication? New tests? Something that breaks the unbearable status quo. She does not want to be held back. My role as GP is ambiguous. My role of holding can be interpreted as holding her back. I don't buy into the romantic fantasy of an ongoing relationship in which the patient is satisfied solely with the comfort of 'being held' by a GP who knows her well, though this can certainly help. In fact, as a grassroot-practitioner, in my encounters with patients, I am often faced with alternative narratives – of restitution, of chaos and of quest (Frank, 2004).

Wendy

On a night shift in Out of Hours, I was called to a dramatic escalation in a different practice area. The patient, let's call her Wendy, had a long history of pelvic uro-gynaecological trouble and a catheter had been inserted to provide a solution. She could not bear this foreign body inside her body, and she also could not bear her dysfunctional bladder. I asked about her GP. She described him as her rock. I know him: he is part of a dying breed of GPs who is embedded within his community and who holds personal knowledge of his patients gathered over a lifetime of working there. He is caring, he is present in local networks and sits on regional committees. I am sure he had a wise opinion on what will work in her best interest. But here and now, in the middle of the night, she wanted the big escape, a referral to the gynaecology unit, even knowing that there will not be this level of trust and familiarity with her situation.

One part of my role as a GP is trying to help the ones I cannot help. This is not mentioned in the official GP curriculum but is commonplace in hidden, street-level GP-bureaucrat curriculum. And this place of intractability is more quickly reached and more common than officially portrayed in the scenarios of evidence based medicine that inform policy and medical examinations.

The insect trying to escape from a glass jar containing sticky lemonade

In this instance, the situation reminds me of observing an insect trying to escape from being stuck in lemonade in a glass. The insect is climbing up, reaches the edge of the glass, and slides down again. Except that as Wendy's GP, I am not an independent, detached observer monitoring the futile attempts of the poor creature. I am part of the situation. I wonder whether as the GP, I am situated with her in the lemonade or further up, towards the rim of the glass. I can predict that Debbie and Wendy will be disappointed if and when they are finally seen by yet another specialist.

Complex holding work is not a romantic steady state; it oscillates between being the problem and the solution and is, like any relationship, a stable unstable steady state.

The complexity of holding work includes sudden twists, flashbacks and bursts of relational violence. There is an in-built asymmetry in the doctor-patient relationship. The ethical stance of curiosity in the hermeneutic window includes openness to change and different ways of interpreting the current status quo. Complex holding work does not have a linear trajectory, it is a spiral of loops with triggering events. We have included Debbie and Wendy as 'live cases' who clearly illustrate the ongoing dramatic nature of holding work with its uncertain outcomes. A fellow GP once received a thank you card from a patient with the inscription 'Thank you for putting up with all my shit over the years' (Tomlinson, J. personal communication, 2024).

Sarah

Sarah is 37 years and very frustrated with being disabled by the intractable fatigue that has held her back for nearly two years. It is not just the brain fog, it is also the sensation of her throat closing, of painful joints and visceral responses to certain smells and sounds. Her senses have become too sensitive, and many organ systems have become equally unpredictable. Her physical functions have become unreliable, her body's machinery and functions no longer operate silently in the background. She wants to reset to the state she was in before her presumed COVID infection. She wants the nightmare to end. She wants things to stop, the fatigue to go.

The first time we met, she came with a lot of bottled-up frustration. She told me about what had been said to her, that she had seen an endocrinologist privately, who sent her back to the GP with a long list of specialist tests – requests to check levels of minerals, enzymes, and hormones in her body. These tests are impossible to order in General Practice. They are expensive. If she pays for them privately, they will cost her £2,000. So, she is back to see the GP. She wants (a) to get to a more suitable state of being and (b) to find a final answer to her predicament.

Overwhelmed by both the emotional impact of the plea to end her ordeal and the size of the task, I asked her to come back with a detailed account and timeline of her problems. I promised to be in a more receptive state than I was then, in my role as 'duty doctor.' Indeed, the next encounter took a different direction. Sarah brought the carefully formatted printout with the list of all her problems. I sat next to her and together, we went through the long litany of symptoms.

There was space. We looked together at the list and condensed it down into two specific referrals to specialists and the task to build a story together. Once we had done that, we agreed to write the referrals together. So, we moved together to the computer. I went over with her carefully what is reasonable to expect from, for example, an ENT consultation and what she would not get. I told her that as her GP I will be with her in the long run. The act of sitting together and dealing with her problem in a different spatial but also relational configuration moved the consultation into the realm of finding and creating meaning. For me, the clinician, it needed both a different mind frame, and also a different physical stance. From face to face to side by side. 'From face-to-face to side-by-side' – consultation models from the 1980s talked about moving from a confrontational space to a co-active one (Horton, 2011). But the inner change in how I position myself as a practitioner parallels that physical shift: I have moved into a hermeneutic stance (see Figure 5.2).

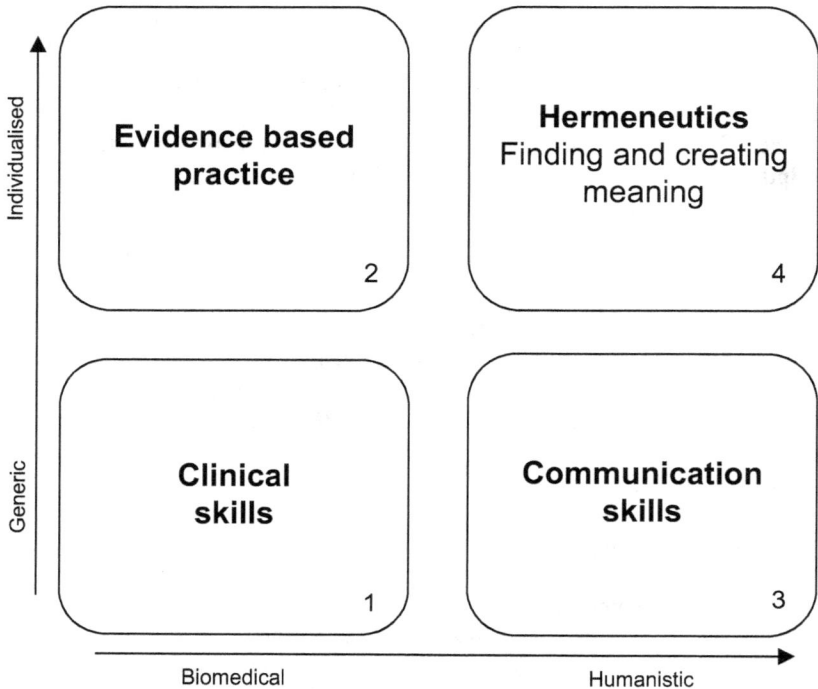

Figure 5.2 The Hermeneutic Window (Shah et al., 2020).

Gareth

Gareth's wife contacts the surgery. She is very concerned about him. He is deeply depressed, does not want to do anything. He is not excited any more about things he used to enjoy. There is no oomph in him. A year ago, he tried to take his life and afterwards, he spent time in the mental health unit, then he was looked after by the home treatment team. Now, he has been discharged from the mental health team, but he feels just as hopeless and numb as before. I invite the couple to come in to see me together. The wife does the talking. His eyes look tearful, but he has an ectropion, that causes his lower eyelid to sag away from the eye, and his eyes to constantly stream. Gareth's wife tells me that he has no energy, he often just stays in his chair all day. She worries about him. They do not go out because he has mentioned thoughts of jumping off a cliff or drowning in the sea. I notice the dirt under his fingernails, the calluses on his hands. They are the hands of somebody who has done manual work all his life. They tell me he had a garage, but he had to give it up. Now he is gradually selling the tools on e-Bay. Losing his garage, which for him is so much more than a garage, affects him profoundly. Also, depression runs in the family, I hear.

We talk about men and sheds, about the meaning of work, about identity, about craft, about a place. The conversation gathers flow, and he becomes more animated.

Practitioner as witness
Practitioner's biographical function
Practitioner's use of self

Intuition in partnership with evidence
How do I sense this?
How do I use the different ways of knowing?

Hermeneutic window

Narrative practice
Emotional engagement and connection
Authenticity and curiosity
Relational ethical framework

Exploring professionalism
What is my role here?
What assumptions am I making?
How do my own experiences affect the interaction?

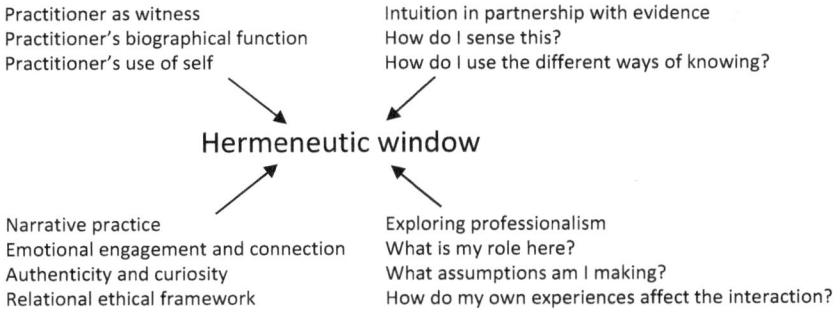

Figure 5.3 The Hermeneutic Window as Reciprocal Space (Shah et al., 2021).

What is expected from a molecule, from a tablet that will be swallowed once or twice a day, from a 'swallowing cure'? Would a 'talking cure' help?

I mention my father and how retirement affected his sense of self. The conversation brought memories of my father back. In this phase of his life, we went to a sports event together and his lack of passion hurt me deeply. He also had lost his oomph, his mojo. Not long after this event he died, and my own narrative interpretation of the cause of death was that he lost his relationship with life and let himself go. I can see a different space opening in the conversation with Gareth and his wife, a hermeneutic space (see Figure 5.3). We start to talk about social places (men's sheds) and things one can do that don't include the act of swallowing tablets. We talk about fitness, and the consultation moves to Gareth's wife's painful joints. She does not want him to leave the house alone in his current state. They ask when they can see me again.

The hermeneutic window as a reciprocal space

The hermeneutic window is a reciprocal space. It works in both dimensions and needs input from patient and clinician. It requires attentiveness and being *present*. It is a bilateral or multilateral space. As such it can be more a 'mind-frame' (like in the film 'Matrix' when Neo is offered a choice of the red pill – the truth about man's enslavement to machines- or the blue pill – a return to ignorance) than a concept like Prochazka's cycle of change or Kuebler-Ross' stages of grief. It is not a static map. It can open psychedelic opportunities, entry to the warren of the white rabbit in Alice's wonderland and we end up banging our heads against a brick wall. The hermeneutic window can be only a mirror, even a distorting mirror. What it does is invite other dimensions to sit alongside mainstream decision-making, or, in another paradigm, invites the right brain hemisphere to connect with the subject matter in a different way (McGilchrist, 2019). This may happen for my own sake (to add another way of connecting or doing the task) or for the sake of the patient. It works both ways and has huge potential.

Healthcare is (and always has been) a human social activity. This means relational aspects of care, where meanings are generated and inter-subjectivity is the landscape, will be ever-present alongside technical aspects. As technicians we are tasked with attempting to understand bodily processes and intervene, where possible, to alleviate suffering and potential suffering that arises from pathological processes. It is this aspect that receives the most attention (for very good reasons) in our medical training. Here we act as biomedical scientist-technicians identifying diseases and prescribing remedies.

But the technician doctor model cannot capture the relational aspects of care that stalk the doctor-patient encounter. The further away we are from acute presentations and time-limited interventions, the greater the encroachment of relationships. When dealing with chronic conditions, unexplained symptoms, and mental health/ distress, we are more immersed in inter-subjective meaning making. This is not only unavoidable, but arguably our choice of hermeneutic scaffolding will have a bigger impact on patient level outcomes than our choice of technical interventions. This is particularly so when there is a significant mental health component (see, for example, (Budd & Hughes, 2009; Cooper, 2008; Drury, 2014; Wampold, 2015).

Entering the hermeneutic window

The importance of relational aspects of healthcare has been known about for decades. In a follow-up meta-analysis of how doctor-patient communication affected outcomes, Stewart (1995) noted that the quality of communication during history-taking and management also affects outcomes such as frequency of visits, emotional health, and symptom resolution. The manner in which a physician communicates with a patient (even while gathering information) influenced how often, and if at all, a patient will return to that same physician. Chipidza et al. (2015) concluded that trust, knowledge, regard and loyalty are the four elements that underpin the doctor-patient relationship, and the nature of this relationship has a significant impact on patient outcomes. Furthermore, the quality of communication between doctor and patient involves assessment of the doctor's willingness to include a patient in the decision-making process, to provide a patient with information, and to ask a patient about his or her explanatory model of illness (Evans et al., 1987; Kleinman et al., 1978).

But what does this academic insight look and 'feel' like in the busy time-challenged consulting room? It is difficult (and undesirable) to give a systematised, process model for the relational space within which meaning is generated. Unlike diagnostic/ treatment process guidelines, relational knowing is non-linear. When we take relational aspects of care seriously nothing can save us from the messiness of real-life encounters that go beyond the intellectual and are charged with emotional energy. It could even be argued that technical aspects of care can function as a defence against having to engage with these human aspects that become increasingly difficult to compartmentalise as we stray into chronic and multi-morbidity complexity.

Here is a real person (and/or their important others) who is suffering sitting in front of you in the consulting room. They have just explained how hopeless they feel and you are, and have been, at a loss as to how you should intervene. What are your options? Can you confide in your uncertainty? Should you conjure up another technical procedure, perhaps alter an existing prescription or try a new one? Should you just make a referral so that someone else can take this problem on? Will that actually prevent or reduce how often this patient attends? Should you engage in a conversation about how they 'feel'? How long might that take given that you have a large caseload to get through this morning? Can you free your mind sufficiently to really *be present* with this patient for the time you have and get that argument you had with your partner this morning out of your head? In the everyday world of emotional turbulence, the temptation to step away and retreat from this maelstrom into the embodiment of the scientist-technician is understandable.

We want to suggest that such a solution may appear to provide short-term relief for the professional but may actually make your job as a doctor more difficult in the long-term. We want to invite you to step through the hermeneutic window and allow that inter-subjectivity into the room in a conscious and aware manner. Understanding the chemical constituents of an apple will be no substitute for biting into it and letting your taste buds be stimulated, so you experience the apple rather than just learn about it. We want doctors, particularly primary care doctors, to be alive to the relational and contextual aspects of being a doctor. A very simple starting point is to be aware of how you are 'positioning yourself' as a practitioner: in other words, to ask yourself the question 'What is my role with this person, right here, right now?' And maybe to include a discussion of how the patient sees your role in the consultation.

You may feel abandoned by theory (Rycroft, 2004). You may find yourself wading through the 'swampy lowlands' of practice. Can you take the risk to enter the psychic space where you have to hang the saviour complex that many (most?) doctors have had drummed into them by years of training and media flattery, on the door next to your metaphorical (or literal) white coat, roll up your sleeve and prepare yourself for some relational toiling. It may seem more difficult than it really is. It may involve some de-learning, a release from disciplinary edicts like moving from classical to jazz, where improvisation and riffing on a theme become foregrounded. Now we can be open to how people, families, and even communities come with their own sense of what they need, their own readiness, their own agendas, and their own willingness to participate in particular ways.

Sometimes when we stop trying so hard to be the possessors of cure knowledge and 'let go' of our expectations of ourselves as doctors, we relate in a way which has a potential to be more therapeutic. In facing our limits, we are more likely to honour the extraordinary in the ordinary. People come with their best and their worst. They may conflict, contradict, be stubborn, despair, disagree, refuse to follow advice, be consensual, amicable, agreeable, hopeful, positive, complaint. There is no reason to imagine the relational space of the consulting room can be expunged from all we find in the relational joys and miseries of our personal lives.

Frameworks for the hermeneutic window

There are many meaning making frameworks that can help us conceptualise and contextualise this hermeneutic space. But we cannot see, feel, weigh, calibrate, and calculate standard deviations for how I came up with those sentences. We cannot escape subjectivity in understanding subjectivity. We cannot discover the 'truth' about why I typed a particular sentence; we can only create a framework to explain that from a limited number of available systems of knowledge that we have been exposed to. Our choice of explanatory framework has profound consequences. A few of frameworks from the psychotherapy world come to mind that may help us be relationally present in particular ways.

Narrative medicine/therapy

Narrative approaches understand that our world of meaning is made of stories that that we internalise about ourselves and our context. We hold many stories that can be influenced by our histories, relationships and media we have been exposed to. Everyone develops unique ways of understanding and storying their lives, which are fluid and changeable. Narrative approaches seek to be a respectful and non-blaming approach, which centre people as the experts in their own lives and attempt to engage with their subjectivity from that starting point.

Narrative practice is founded on the idea that the stories that we tell about ourselves are not private and individual but are a social achievement. The idea of involving others to listen in therapeutic conversations is not new. Within the tradition of family therapy, teams of professionals often listened to families from behind a one-way screen and then made various interventions depending upon the model of therapy. Tom Andersen (1987) challenged the anonymity of these teams of professionals and began a range of explorations into the use of reflecting work. Michael White (1995) brought these ideas of outsider witnesses into a variety of therapeutic practices.

Narrative approaches place a particular significance on maintaining a stance of curiosity and asking questions to which you genuinely do not know the answers. Our questions and conjectures will influence the potential stories that will be expanded for further reflection. There are many cross-roads, intersections, paths, and tracks to choose from. At the beginning of an inter-subjective journey, we are not sure where it will end, nor what will be discovered.

There is a strand of narrative therapy sometimes called 'outsider witness practice.' This approach is used as a means of helping people see and bear witness to their own worth and identities (White, 1995). An audience (of potential outsider witnesses – such as the doctor) is invited to listen and reflect on the patient's story in that patient's own terms and language. The role of the audience is to help the person make space for an alternative story to emerge. Importantly, the outsider witness does not provide 'expert' commentary or offer advice.

The outsider witness process is a practice of 'acknowledgment' in which some aspects of a person's story 'resonate' at that human inter-subjective level with the listener. With the case of Gareth above, the doctor honoured his predicament by allowing himself to react to the ripples of storied memories from his own life. In the doctor recounting a story about his seeing his father lose his mojo, his oomph, a type of connection through shared meaningful human stories helped the patient and his partner 'feel' that the doctor was present, hearing and feeling something of their situation. That sense of someone, with social authority, 'getting it,' created a new opportunity for something to move, to rekindle a lost aspect of the patient's potential future story.

Social constructivism is the view that learning occurs through social interaction and each person's understanding of how the world works is shaped through the knowledge that gets passed to them by the social interactions they are exposed to. Social constructivism has many roots and bifurcations but is thought to have been developed into a coherent theory by Soviet psychologist Lev Vygotsky (1896–1934). Vygotsky believed that knowledge is not a copy of an objective reality but rather the result of the mind selecting, making sense of, and then mentally recreating experiences. Knowledge is thus the result of interactions between both subjective and environmental factors. In other words, it is 'constructed' out of the variety of experiences we are exposed to and moulded by our subjective interpretations of the significance of these for the individual. Social constructivism is closely related to narrative approaches.

When we notice someone's capacity for survival buried within the stories of suffering, we find a sub-plot waiting to be explored. We may then have a role in helping construct a version of the patient's story that goes beyond witnessing, acknowledging and dignifying a patient's experiences. We may have a role in helping them notice aspects of their life and story that become buried under the weight of the story of suffering. It may be helpful to remember that stories of suffering are also stories of survival. We may have a role in recognising people's capacity to survive and keep going, even if it's just to hold that knowledge in our own minds.

Hugh Middleton (2023) has written about the power of a social network to shape what meanings we internalise. Relationships with patients and their close associates has an essential role to play in subsequent outcomes. How a person makes sense of their suffering, changes how a person experiences their suffering. Changing ideas change people. Doctors are often important conduits in shaping how people understand, experience and deal with their health-related anxieties and problems.

An acutely distressed person might generate a range of responses: 'You are obviously having a hard time and deserve a little more care and attention,' 'I am concerned about their risk to themselves and so will organise a mental health act assessment,' 'I will make an urgent referral and start you on an antidepressant as this is the clinical pathway we follow under such circumstances,' 'I don't know how I would have handled it if this happened to me, how did you even manage to get up and get in to see me this morning?'. None of those are right or wrong responses, but each is loaded with different implications and consequences for how this person's care journey will unfold and for what aspect of their story will be highlighted and thickened.

Containment and holding: in psychoanalytic theory, the notion of containment or holding is about the analyst's ability to hold or contain the patient's anxiety without needing to reject, react, or otherwise by-pass the feelings it evokes in the analyst. It is the capacity to sit with and tolerate the patient's distress – something doctors have to be able to find a way to accomplish in everyday practice. Wilfred

Bion's (1962) concept of the container/contained and Donald Winnicott's (1958) concept of holding are two notions that have had a profound influence on the development of psychotherapeutic approaches to people in distress. It derives from observing how an infant who is overwhelmed by distress and having no context to understand the experience, is held and soothed by the parent, who thus creates a safe context for the child to be distressed and where psychological growth and development can then occur.

Holding and containing a patient's distress allows an opportunity for that distress to be experienced without necessitating a retreat into the infantile fantasy (whether by the patient or the doctor) that all suffering can be magicked away. Holding and containing just means being able to sit with pain and discomfort without panic and plotting an escape route. It is not to do with whether or not you take out your prescription pad (although you might). It is to do where you are in your own mind, so that you recognise and resist the impulse to eliminate pain (your own mental pain) at any cost.

Conclusion

Hermeneutic approaches are particularly relevant in consultations with patients with chronic pain, medically unexplained symptoms and mental health issues such as depression. Although falling back on 'just another referral' or 'just another blood test' may save time in the short-term, we argue that engaging with meaning making can help witness, acknowledge and dignify suffering and can catalyse new perspectives, understanding and narrative for both patient and doctor. Simple interventions can be transformative. In the midst of the complexity and apparent chaos of such presentations, when the limitations of 'doctor as saviour' are becoming apparent, simply reflecting on the question 'What is my role with this person, what do they want my role to be and what could it potentially be?' signals that the practitioner has entered the hermeneutic window.

References

Andersen, T. (1987). The reflecting team: Dialogue and meta-dialogue in clinical work. *Family process, 26*(4), 415–428.

Atkin, P. (2023). *Some of us just fall: On nature and not getting better*. Hachette UK.

Barnard, R., Spooner, S., Hubmann, M., Checkland, K., Campbell, J., & Swinglehurst, D. (2024). The hidden work of general practitioners: An ethnography. *Social Science & Medicine, 350*, 116922.

Bion, W. (1962). Learning from experience. Heinemann.

Budd, R., & Hughes, I. (2009). The Dodo Bird Verdict—controversial, inevitable and important: A commentary on 30 years of meta-analyses. *Clinical Psychology & Psychotherapy: An International Journal of Theory & Practice, 16*(6), 510–522.

Chipidza, F, Wallwork, R., & Stern, T. (2015). Impact of the doctor-patient relationship. *The Primary Care Companion for CNS Disorders, 17*(5), 27354.

Cocksedge, S., Greenfield, R., Nugent, G., & Chew-Graham, C. (2011). Holding relationships in primary care: A qualitative exploration of doctors' and patients' perceptions. *British Journal of General Practice, 61*(589), e484–e491.

Cooper, M. (2008). *Essential research findings in counselling and psychotherapy: The facts are friendly*. Sage Publishing.

Drury, N. (2014). Mental health is an abominable mess: Mind and nature is a necessary unity. *New Zealand Journal of Psychology, 43*(1), 5–17.

Evans, B., Kiellerup, F., Stanley, R., Burrows, G., & Sweet, B. (1987). A communication skills programme for increasing patients' satisfaction with general practice consultations. *British Journal of Medical Psychology, 60*(4), 373–378.

Frank, A. W. (2004). Asking the right question about pain: Narrative and phronesis. *Literature and Medicine, 23*(2), 209–225.

Horton, R. (2011). Offline: Face to face, side by side. *The Lancet, 377*(9773), 1224.

Kleinman, A., Eisenberg, L., & Good, B. (1978). Culture, illness, and care: Clinical lessons from anthropologic and cross-cultural research. *Annals of Internal Medicine, 88*(2), 251–258. https://doi.org/10.7326/0003-4819-88-2-251

Lipsky, M. (1980). *Street-level bureaucracy: Dilemmas of the individual in public service*. Russell Sage Foundation.

McGilchrist, I. (2019). *The master and his emissary: The divided brain and the making of the western world*. Yale University Press.

Middleton, H. (2023). *Toxic interactions and the social geography of psychosis: Reflections on the epidemiology of mental disorder*. Taylor & Francis.

Rycroft, P. (2004). When theory abandons us–wading through the 'swampy lowlands' of practice. *Journal of Family Therapy, 26*(3), 245–259.

Shah, R., Clarke, R., Ahluwalia, S., & Launer, J. (2020). Finding meaning in the consultation: Introducing the hermeneutic window. *British Journal of General Practice, 70*(699), 502–503.

Shah, R., Clarke, R., Ahluwalia, S., & Launer, J. (2021). Finding meaning in the consultation: Working in the hermeneutic window. *British Journal of General Practice, 71*(707), 282–283.

Stewart, M. (1995). Effective physician-patient communication and health outcomes: A review. *Canadian Medical Association Journal, 152*(9), 1423.

Wampold, B. (2015). *The great psychotherapy debate: The evidence for what makes psychotherapy work*. Routledge.

White, M. (1995). Reflecting teamwork as definitional ceremony. In *Re-authoring Lives: Interviews and Essays* (pp. 172–198). Dulwich Centre Publications.

Winnicott, D. (1958). *Collected papers: Through paediatrics to psychoanalysis*. Routledge.

6   Hermeneutics – an ethical and philosophical perspective

Paquita de Zulueta and John Spicer

Introduction

There is a clear paradox in modern healthcare. Despite increased sophistication in technology, diagnostics and therapeutics, public dissatisfaction is rising, costs are escalating and the healthcare professional workforce is showing alarming levels of burnout and demoralisation in the UK and elsewhere. The 'soul' of medicine, including that of general practice, is being sucked out (Shah & Foell, 2024).

Clinicians who endeavour to practise kind and careful care, to offer compassion and genuine caregiving, struggle in an industrialised, bureaucratised system that becomes progressively more dehumanising. It is dehumanising in two ways: firstly by removing the human from many interactions and forcing patients to be 'processed' like widgets, and secondly by constraining healthcare professionals to frequently behave as automatons on a factory line, rather than as professionals.

Taylorism, 'the scientific management of organisations' (Taylor, 1911), which advocates an engineering machine-like model for human systems, was established over 100 years ago, yet still lives on, now enhanced by commercialisation, digitalisation and 'remote' systems of care. Industrialisation and unbridled scientific materialism in healthcare lead to reification or objectification of humans and the instrumentalisation of relationships (Honneth, 2005). The combination of heavy reliance on evidence based medicine (EBM) and rigidly applied bureaucratisation is termed scientific bureaucratic medicine, or SBM (Harrison et al., 2002).

SBM is considered incompatible with dynamic, complex illness and with the nuances of relational care (Reeve, 2010; Sweeney et al., 1998) and is responsible for much of the alienation and distress experienced by carers and patients alike (Heath, 2016). This alienation is felt particularly in primary care, but also in secondary care. We do not deny the gains that the scientific approach has made in modern medicine, or its usefulness, but we need to recognise its limits as well as the harms that can result if the lived experience of both patients and practitioners are ignored or eclipsed. The success of modern medical science has made it hard to see that medicine is, at its core, about healing relationships between persons and not simply a scientific investigation of biological organisms (Svenaeus, 2022). This is where hermeneutics comes to the rescue – the study of how we interpret the world around us and make sense of it. It can also be thought of as the art of understanding and making oneself understood.

DOI: 10.4324/9781003517665-6

Hermeneutics – a challenge to scientific materialism

Hermeneutic thinkers believe that all understanding is the interpretive act of integrating particulars – words, signs, events into a meaningful whole and that these then become part of our inner mental world. It is our fundamental way of 'being-in-the-world' – *dasein* – a term coined by Heidegger (Heidegger, 1996). Hermeneutics challenges the belief, prevalent in modern day, that 'real' knowledge consists in quantification – the scientific numerical description of the world – and that objective truth requires an impersonal, theoretical stance. Instead, quite radically, the hermeneutical stance proposes that our primary mode of perception is practical and intrinsically connected to the context of our experience, our desires and our interests.

The three central claims of hermeneutics are:

1 The 'engaged self' is fundamentally connected to the world and to other people. Consciousness itself is shaped by the way we inhabit the world.
2 Hermeneutic thinkers believe that we need to redefine 'objective' truth as something we take part in rather than observe from a distance and that our historically formed conceptual lenses allow us meaningful access to reality.
3 The only way we can experience the world as meaningful is through interpretation. Language helps us to express and interpret our perceptions.

When we consider these claims, it is useful to juxtapose them with the philosophical framework of 'phenomenology,' which is the study of conscious experience 'that views cognition as embodied, focuses on subjective experience and provides a robust existential account of selfhood.' It is highly suited to understanding the experience of illness (Carel, 2012).

A phenomenological understanding shows that both the science and art of medicine are grounded in 'the lifeworld' – the world of everyday human experience. The philosopher and mathematician Edmund Husserl (1839–1938) considered the lifeworld to be the foundation of meaning for all human existence (Husserl, 1970).

Schwartz and Wiggins (1985) argue that medical practice is only intelligible 'when its moorings in a fundamental domain of human experience are clarified and delineated.' The natural sciences offer precision and predictability at the expense of discarding experiences of illness that are crucial to helping patients recover and flourish. We argue that ignoring this lived experience results in a form of injustice – called hermeneutic injustice that we expand upon below. Engel's biopsychosocial model (Engel, 1977), albeit redressing some gaps, does not counter the reliance of medicine on data.

The real problem with the biomedical model is its abstractness (the word is derived from the Latin *abstrahere*, to draw away from) or reductionism. This 'spirit of abstraction,' prevalent since the rise of modern science in the sixteenth and seventeenth centuries, means that certain aspects of reality are excluded in the pursuit of conceptual precision. These powerful abstractions, on which technologies are based, enable us to make precise inferences and predictions. But reductionism can also lead to the 'fallacy of misplaced concreteness,' a phrase coined by the philosopher-mathematician

Alfred North Whitehead (Whitehead, 1925, p. 52). Ordinary lived experiences are dismissed or deprioritised as irrelevant or 'subjective.' Indeed, the natural sciences have set aside so many facets of human existence in order to reach precision and exactitude that arguably they retain little of what makes people truly human. If this is the only lens or window through which we see the patient-as-ill, then, inevitably it will dehumanise (Beresford, 2010; Evans, 2003).

McWhinney (1997) comments on how this abstraction underlies one of the paradoxes of the doctor-patient relationship: as modern medicine has become technologically more successful, dissatisfaction has increased. He conjectures that the rise in 'pathographies' (personal accounts of illness) is a response to the eclipse of the patient's voice and their lived experience, a view endorsed by Frank (1995, 2004) and Mishler (2005).

Hermeneutics, however, offers a comprehensive, holistic context which incorporates the rich complexity of human life. Acknowledging and restoring the primacy of the lifeworld will combat the spirit of abstraction and help to resolve the ongoing crisis in healthcare. Hermeneutics has radical importance for revealing what is happening between clinicians and patients in modern healthcare generally. Its devaluation in clinical practice creates tensions and fissures; and often misery and confusion.

Medical consultations, dialogue and the 'lifeworld'

Mishler's qualitative analysis of medical consultations (1984) applies Habermas' critique of the modern world's technocratic consciousness (1970) to the clinical encounter, whereby the patient's lifeworld is transformed into a technical-medical problem: 'the voice of medicine.' Habermas' theory of communicative action (1984), describes two kinds of rationality: firstly, communicative, or value rationality which inhabits the 'lifeworld,' is orientated towards understanding, and is underpinned by moral considerations, and secondly, purposive rationality which inhabits 'the system.' The latter represents the scientific attitude reliant on abstract rules and stripped of context or moral dimensions. Habermas' proposal for communication allows for respectful dialogue such that an open space can be created within which mutual understanding and common purpose can be negotiated – a valuable guide for conversation between clinicians and patients (Hazzard et al., 2013). Epstein's (2012) concept of 'shared minds,' although not described from a phenomenological viewpoint, chimes with this form of dialogical communication. Attention to the patient's lifeworld creates trust early on in the relationship (Norberg Boysen et al., 2017).

In his study, Mishler shows how the 'voice of medicine' (medical science/ the system) fragments and suppresses the lifeworld leading to inhumane and even ineffective care. Barry et al. (2001) expanded this research by collecting data from patient interviews, doctor interviews and transcribed consultations. They found four communication patterns to emerge:

1 *Mutual lifeworld* when both patient and doctor are engaged with the lifeworld.
2 *Strictly lifeworld* when both patient and doctor use the voice of medicine exclusively.

3 *Lifeworld blocked.*
4 *Lifeworld ignored* – when the patient uses the voice of the lifeworld, but it is blocked or ignored.

Close analysis shows that these categories are not so clearcut and there can be a shift within the consultation. Barry concludes that Mischler's theory of the dialectical struggle between the voice of medicine and the voice of the lifeworld is a useful way of looking at doctor-patient communications. Unsurprisingly, the need to be listened to, understood and treated as whole unique human beings had greater prominence for those with chronic or debilitating conditions. But many would argue that the current structural aspects of the healthcare system are not conducive to lifeworld-centred care.

In the research by Barry et al., it was noted that some of the 'lifeworld consultations' had taken longer than ten minutes, but several had not, with an average consultation time of 8mins. So perhaps time is not the crucial factor, although no doubt it plays a part. Perhaps it is more about attention and intention – a willingness to listen and engage with the patient's lifeworld and narrative.

Blending of horizons in the clinical encounter

Clinicians' behaviour is shaped by their professional training, experience, and expectations. Through increased self-awareness and by listening with an open mind, setting aside acquired conventional and social meanings, clinicians can better engage with the patient's 'horizon,' leading to a 'blending of horizons' (Husserl, 1970). However, this does not mean colonising the patient's lifeworld; the separateness, or alterity, of the patient remains intact. This alterity is key to the philosophy of Paul Ricoeur (Russo, 2021) and Emmanuel Levinas. Indeed, for Levinas, ethics is founded on the experience of the encounter with the Other. The epiphany of recognising the Other's 'face' is a phenomenon in which the other person's proximity and distance are both strongly felt, creating a non-negotiable ethical responsibility. 'I am called to apprehend the world from the Other's perspective and to respond. The face has authority without power and creates an ethical force' (Clifton-Soderstrom, 2003; Levinas, 1961).

Embodiment, touch and embodied consciousness

Key to phenomenology is the recognition that we inhabit and act in the lifeworld as embodied subjects. At the concrete level of lived experience, the mind and body are one. Movement displays our basic intentionality. The body is the core of one's existence and the basis for any interaction with the world (Merleau-Ponty, 1945, 2002). Our living flesh is how we perceive our surroundings, move towards desired goals, and interact with others, resonating with their moods and intentions (Leder, 2016). Illness, particularly chronic illness, is a disruption of the lived body, rather than dysfunction of the biological body, and redefines the relationship of the person to the world and to self. Leder (2021) describes how adaptation to illness always has an embodied dimension, but this can be overlooked when there is an excessive focus on psychological resilience. The importance of touch in healing encounters should not be overlooked (de Zulueta, 2020).

Ethical implications for clinical practice

Creative capacity

For simple acute, self-limiting problems a biomedical approach may be sufficient (Barry et al., 2001; Savage & Armstrong, 1990), but often it will not suffice, particularly in the context of chronic disease, prolonged disability and conditions which defy conventional diagnosis. As Kleinman (1988, p. 17) observes, practitioners can find chronic illness 'messy, and threatening' and the drive for quantification and objectivity 'can make a shambles of the care of the chronically ill.'

Toombs (1987), reflecting on her own experience of illness (multiple sclerosis), proposes that the reason communication between doctors and patients is often fraught and unsatisfactory is because of a fundamental disagreement, or incommensurability, in how illness is conceived and understood. There is a significant gap between the way physicians generally think about illness – as an abstracted, decontextualised manifestation of disease – and how it is experienced by the patient, in particular how it affects his/her everyday life and function. Toombs describes in vivid detail the existential perspective of living with chronic illness. She talks about loss: the perception of loss of wholeness and bodily integrity, loss of certainty, freedom and control, and loss of a hitherto familiar world. The malfunctioning or painful body can be experienced as alien and unreliable: 'illness disrupts the fundamental unity between body and self.'

Carel (2012) also advocates for the phenomenological approach as it can offer a 'thick account' of the patient experience. As she says:

> The materialism and mechanistic view of the body implicit in the medical model are of limited use when offered to patients as a framework for understanding their illness experience.

Carel argues that biomedical approaches neglect the loss of agency or incapacity that characterise the experience of illness; compared to phenomenology, which offers a 'relational account' of the lived person, including her daily activities, goals and interactions with the environment and social world. She describes how illness leads to a changed perception of space and time, lost abilities, and the development of adaptability – it changes the way in which people experience life, influencing identity and leading to a change in values and priorities.

Carel proposes that people have creative capacity to adapt in the face of illness and to re-imagine life in a new context. Reeve (2017) further develops this concept by putting forward the idea of the 'creative self' who can adapt in response to illness. Carel advocates for the recognition of 'health within illness' (Lindsey, 1996), by finding new meaning in illness, and developing an adaptive and creative response – a 'reconciliation.' This process can take many years and can be supported by a clinician who can help their patient identify and develop their adaptive and creative capabilities. Carel offers a 'phenomenological toolkit' to help achieve this adaptation.

Sticking to a strictly biomedical paradigm in medicine in which the lifeworld is sidelined fails to harness and build upon individual creative capacity; therefore this has ethical implications that are not commonly discussed.

Suffering and the eclipse of the lifeworld

Suffering (Figure 6.1) is a neglected topic in medicine, yet the relief of suffering should be its fundamental goal and the core of its ethics (Cassell, 1982, 2004; Kleinman, 1988). Medical treatment may fail to alleviate suffering and may even become a source of suffering in its own right. By ignoring or blocking the patient's lifeworld, doctors create additional suffering for the patient, as revealed by the many stories of patienthood (Carel, 2008; Frank, 1995, 2004; Sweeney et al., 2009).

Cassell, in his description of suffering, adopts a different conceptual approach, yet he echoes much of what Toombs and Carel say, and emphasises the complex and personal experience of illness and the many ways in which is causes suffering. Frank, referring to Habermas' theory, calls for a 'pedagogy of suffering,' foregrounding the body's vulnerability and pain.

The phenomenological conceptualisation of suffering and pain within embodiment offers a powerful alternative to dualistic theories and mechanistic understanding of the body (Bueno-Gómez, 2017). Phenomenology can also provide an understanding of the placebo effect that challenges classical medical explanations. A hermeneutic stance might therefore help clinicians to alleviate suffering.

Epistemic privilege and epistemic injustice in medicine

We have already drawn a distinction between knowledge (*episteme* in Aristotelian terms) and interpreted knowledge. The notion of *episteme* matters in terms of how we consider another aspect of hermeneutics in medicine. The word is derived from

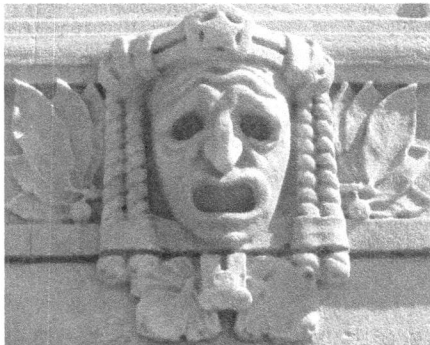

Figure 6.1 Mask of Suffering (Ellgaard, 2008; Photo).

the Greek, meaning 'knowledge' in ancient times, though interestingly it is construed as 'science' in modern language. *Episteme* is often allied with *techne* (craft) and *phronesis* (practical wisdom), all of which are held to be core components of medical professionalism. As we have shown, biomedical knowledge of diseases is often insufficient to alleviate suffering when it does not include the patient's lived experience and the meaning that their illness represents for them. Practitioners, in their endeavour to interpret symptoms and obtain a clinical diagnosis often prioritise the objective body over the lived body of illness, thereby eclipsing vital elements of the patient's experience (Wardrope & Reuber, 2022). Indeed, it may be difficult if not impossible for some individuals to articulate their symptoms in a way that 'fits' the biomedical paradigm.

Privileging the medical voice – epistemic privilege – means that it is taken to be the authoritative one and disadvantages other voices, creating hermeneutical marginalisation. Wardrope argues that the disproportionately high epistemic privilege accorded to medicine results in other voices being systematically disadvantaged and marginalised. He advocates for clinicians to adopt epistemic humility. Epistemic injustice, a term coined by Fricker (2007) describes two forms injustice. Firstly, she describes 'testimonial injustice' to the speaker when '…prejudice on the hearer's part causes him to give less credibility to the speaker than he would otherwise have done.' As clinicians, it is normal practice to choose which parts of our patients' stories to privilege and which to ignore. In a sense, it is what we are trained to do.

Secondly 'hermeneutic injustice' is the injustice caused by people being unable to make sense of certain experiences in their life, owing to a lack of the hermeneutical/interpretive resources required to do so. Sometimes this results from deliberate exclusion from access to resources that might help them to understand what has happened (eg someone living in poverty). Hermeneutic injustice also refers to the interpretive gap between speaker and hearer caused by their differing experiences and knowledge. But there may be situations when dominantly situated knowers refuse to accept the epistemic tools developed by those who are marginally situated – a 'wilful hermeneutical ignorance' (Pohlhaus, 2012). For example, most clinicians may not have had the experience of living with chronic insecurity arising from the threat of violence, abuse or from poverty. They will therefore inevitably find it difficult to understand the experience of patients who are living through such situations. The issue at stake is whether we try to bridge the gap. Authors such as Carel and Kidd (2014) offer practitioners practical means of avoiding epistemic injustice.

Relational care mitigates against epistemic injustice. Within a relational ethics framework, ethical decision making is enmeshed within and dependent upon the practitioner patient relationship (Shah et al., 2023). Its principles are mutual respect; engagement; embodied knowledge; environment; and uncertainty (Pollard, 2015). Pollard argues that interactions between people generate a feeling of responsibility for the other and that it is this which determines the morality of the subsequent action. In other words, the nature of the relationship itself has bearing on the morality or otherwise of clinical decisions. A relationship that incorporates the principles listed above enables the lifeworld of the patient as well as the science to be factored into such decisions. Long-term relationships between clinicians and patients are therefore important. Along with the increasing evidence of better health outcomes where continuity of care is fostered and cherished (Gray et al., 2018; Hansen et al., 2013; Sandvik et al., 2022), the qualities of such relationships can alleviate testimonial and hermeneutic injustice between 'hearers' and 'speakers.'

Case studies 1 and 2: injustice, autonomy and capacity

Case study 1: Mrs B

Mrs B, a woman in her mid-fifties, has poorly controlled diabetes. Several medications have been tried and she has seen three dietitians in the past three years. The practice is incentivised to take part in a quarterly diabetes multidisciplinary team (MDT) meeting in which the most complex 'cases' are discussed. The conclusion of the MDT, attended by Mrs B's GP, the practice clinical pharmacist and diabetes specialist nurse is that she should be started on a twice daily insulin regime. Doing this will mean she will likely be forced to take early retirement from her job as a bus driver. Mrs B's GP invites her to come in and explains what has been proposed and why it is necessary. Mrs B agrees to start treatment.

Case analysis

Epistemic injustice

So far, the practitioners looking after Mrs B have only deployed generic skills (within domains 1 and 3 of the Four Domain Model) – they have followed guidelines and communicated next steps sympathetically to Mrs B. However, because they have not interpreted the evidence in an individualised way for her or attempted to enter her lifeworld, Mrs B is still subject to epistemic injustice. She will retire from work ten years earlier than she was planning to, with all the associated social and financial implications. Entering domain 4, the hermeneutic window likely involves an extended appointment, in which she is asked about her story, about her relationship with food, about her understanding of diabetes and about what matters to her. If this happened, it might surface that Mrs B started comfort eating when she was in an abusive marriage and still subconsciously uses food as an emotional crutch because she is lonely; and that becoming a bus driver means a lot to her because it gave her the financial independence that allowed her to finally end the marriage. This conversation might allow Mrs B to understand her own behaviour better (enhancing her creative capacity) and could also open up other treatment options. Its absence results in a form of epistemic injustice (Shah et al., 2023), which people from socially disadvantaged backgrounds are more likely to be affected by (see also Chapter 7, Social Justice).

Autonomy

In the West, we have a highly individualised view of autonomy compared to more family centred approaches adopted in many countries. Spicer et al. (2021) argue that our decisions are not made in a vacuum and are in fact highly influenced by context and by our relationships, including the relationship between practitioner and patient. Therefore, our current conceptualisation of autonomy may be inadequate.

Let us consider this case in terms of the way in which the clinicians involved in her care have supported Mrs B's autonomous decision making. Although Mrs B has theoretically made an autonomous decision when she agrees to start insulin, it could be argued that in fact she acceded because she wasn't given the opportunity to consider with her clinicians the whole context around her poor sugar control; and to make the connection between her sugar control and her comfort eating. Also, if any of the clinicians involved in her care had an established relationship with her, she might have felt more empowered to ask further questions and perhaps to challenge the decision about starting insulin; and the clinician(s) might have felt more of a sense of responsibility for her overall well being.

Case study 2: Dorothy

Rehan is the family doctor of 83-year-old Dorothy, whom he knows well. She has multiple pathologies causing impaired mobility, and difficulty coping at home, though for the most part she manages fairly well, unassisted by social care provision, which she has repeatedly declined. Rehan sees Dorothy one afternoon after she has 'deteriorated' – there is no clear diagnosis to account for these further mobility issues. Her son is present at the consultation. Despite an active conversation between Rehan and Dorothy as to what should happen next in terms of her care, in particular whether or not she should be admitted to hospital or if a trial of treatment should be attempted at home, Dorothy appears confused and repeatedly defers to her son, saying he 'knows what the best thing to do is…' After some deliberation, her son asks Rehan not to admit his mother to hospital.

Case analysis

Capacity and autonomous decision making

Decisions about treatment are not straightforward in cases like this, where capacity is impaired; and the views of the family may be taken into account even in the absence of a formal power of attorney. Rehan's longstanding relationship with Dorothy means that she has spoken to him several times about her son – and Rehan understands how much she loves and trusts him and how much they went through together after the premature death of Dorothy's husband. In this case, although Rehan's clinical decision might be to admit Dorothy to hospital, taking account of her lifeworld leads to him accepting that a trial of treatment at home is probably more in keeping with her values, particularly her strong drive to remain independent. It also allows him to understand what it would mean for her son if she were admitted to hospital and deteriorated there, becoming incapacitated.

Rehan's relationship with Dorothy formed over many years of caring for her means he feels a moral responsibility towards her. Adopting a hermeneutic stance allows him to grapple with complexity and make a moral decision collaboratively with Dorothy's son, accepting the inherent uncertainty of the situation.

Conclusion

We can envisage hermeneutic and biomedical approaches acting together as in the Chinese concept of yin-yang: an opposite but interconnected, self-perpetuating cycle (Launer, 2019; see also Chapter 10). This concept resonates with the relationship of the right and left brain as described by McGilchrist (2009, 2011). The right brain offers a broad empathic attention that takes in the whole, embedded in a real world context, whereas the left brain adopts a narrowly focused beam of attention, a tendency to see things in parts, abstracted and schematised. The two hemispheres work together, but the right should be the 'master' and the left the 'emissary.' McGilchrist believes that the reverse is now happening and this creates a threat to our flourishing and even our very existence. It mirrors the unfortunate tendency for the biomedical to dominate the phenomenological.

Hermeneutic phenomenology offers a philosophy of medicine that validates medical practice as an interpretive activity with a specific structure and goal: regained health. Arguably it is *the* window of which other perspectives form a part. The crisis in modern medicine can only be overcome if the lifeworld is recognised as the foundation for both medical science and humanistic practice. Failure to do so results in injustice, which may be more marked when patients are not able to advocate for themselves.

Modern medicine progressively abstracts from social context, lived experience, immediate sensory perception, healing touch, and even human language. This abstraction is believed to lead to greater efficiency and efficacy, although that is contestable. At any rate, it carries the risk of being profoundly dehumanising to both patients and caregivers. Structural and ideological aspects of the healthcare system militate against a hermeneutic and humane approach. Something vital is lost in translation. Yet the change in demographics, the increased proportion of complex, chronic patterns of ill health, the increased sophistication of medical diagnostics and treatments, combined with a growing disaffection with modern healthcare, creates an imperative for a different way of attending to illness and health. Time for a paradigm shift.

References

Barry, C., Stevenson, F., Britten, N., Barber, N., & Bradley, C. (2001). Giving voice to the lifeworld. More humane, more effective medical care? A qualitative study of doctor-patient communication in general practice. *Social Science and Medicine, 53*(4), 487–505. https://doi.org/10.1016/s0277-9536(00)00351-8

Beresford, M. (2010). Medical reductionism: Lessons from the great philosophers. *QJM: An International Journal of Medicine, 103*(9), 721–724. https://doi.org/10.1093/qjmed/hcq057

Bueno-Gómez, N. (2017). Conceptualizing suffering and pain. *Philosophy, Ethics, and Humanities in Medicine, 12*(1), 7. https://doi.org/10.1186/s13010-017-0049-5

Carel, H. (2008). *Illness: The cry of the flesh.* Routledge.

Carel, H. (2012). Phenomenology as a resource for patients. *Journal of Medicine and Philosophy, 37*(2), 96–113.

Carel, H., & Kidd, I. (2014). Epistemic injustice in healthcare: A philosophial analysis. *Medicine, Health Care and Philosophy, 17*, 529–540.

Cassell, E. (1982). The nature of suffering and the goals of medicine. *New England Journal of Medicine, 306*(11), 639–645. https://doi.org/10.1056/nejm198203183061104

Cassell, E. (2004). *The nature of suffering and the goals of medicine.* Oxford University Press. https://doi.org/10.1093/acprof:oso/9780195156164.001.0001

Clifton-Soderstrom, M. (2003). Levinas and the patient as other: The ethical foundation of medicine. *The Journal of medicine and philosophy, 28*(4), 447–460.

de Zulueta, P. (2020). Touch matters: COVID-19, physical examination, and 21st century general practice. *British Journal of General Practice, 70*(701), 594–595. https://doi.org/10.3399/bjgp20X713705

Ellgaard, H. (2008). *Dramaten mask 2008a* (Photograph of sculpture by Carl Milles). Wikimedia Commons. https://commons.wikimedia.org/wiki/File:Dramaten_mask_2008a.jpg

Engel, G. (1977). The need for a new medical model: A challenge for biomedicine. *Science, 196*(4286), 129–136.

Epstein, R. (2012). Whole mind and shared mind in clinical decision-making. *Patient Education and Counseling, 90*(2), 200–206. https://doi.org/10.1016/j.pec.2012.06.035

Evans, R. (2003). Patient centred medicine: Reason, emotion, and human spirit? Some philosophical reflections on being with patients. *Medical humanities, 29*(1), 8–14.

Frank, A. (1995). *The wounded storyteller: Body, illness & ethics.* University of Chicago Press.

Frank, A. (2004). *The renewal of generosity: Illness, medicine, and how to live.* University of Chicago Press.

Fricker, M. (2007). *Epistemic injustice: Power and the ethics of knowing.* Oxford University Press.

Gray, D., Sidaway-Lee, K., White, E., Thorne, A., & Evans, P. (2018). Continuity of care with doctors—a matter of life and death? A systematic review of continuity of care and mortality. *BMJ Open, 8*(6), e021161.

Habermas, J. (1970). *Toward a rational society.* Beacon Press.

Habermas, J. (1984). *The theory of communicative action-reason and the rationalization of society* (Vol. 1). Polity Press.

Hansen, A., Halvorsen, P., Aaraas, I., & Førde, O. (2013). Continuity of GP care is related to reduced specialist healthcare use: A cross-sectional survey. *British Journal of General Practice, 63*(612), e482–e489. https://doi.org/10.3399/bjgp13X669202

Harrison, S., Moran, M., & Wood, B. (2002). Policy emergence and policy convergence: the case of 'scientific-bureaucratic medicine' in the United States and United Kingdom *British Journal of Politics and International Relations, 4*, 1–24.

Hazzard, A., Harris, W., & Howell, D. (2013). Taking care: Practice and philosophy of communication in a Critical Care follow-up clinic. *Intensive and Critical Care Nursing, 29*(3), 158–165. https://doi.org/10.1016/j.iccn.2013.01.003

Heath, I. (2016). How medicine has exploited rationality at the expense of humanity: An essay by Iona Heath. *British Medical Journal, 355*, i5705. https://doi.org/10.1136/bmj.i5705

Heidegger, M. (1996). *Being and time*: A Translation of Sein und Zeit. State University of New York Press.

Honneth, A. (2005). *Reification: A recognition-theoretical view. The Tanner lectures on human values*. University of California.

Husserl, E. (1970). *The crisis of European sciences and transcendental phenomenology: An introduction to phenomenological philosophy*. Northwestern University Press.

Kleinman, A. (1988). *The illness narratives: Suffering, healing, and the human condition*. Basic books.

Launer, J. (2019). The Yin and Yang of medical consultations. *Postgraduate Medical Journal, 95*(1128), 575–576. https://doi.org/10.1136/postgradmedj-2019-136947

Leder, D. (2016). *The distressed body: Rethinking illness, imprisonment, and healing*. University of Chicago Press.

Leder, D. (2021). Healing time: The experience of body and temporality when coping with illness and incapacity. *Medicine, Health Care and Philosophy, 24*(1), 99–111. https://doi.org/10.1007/s11019-020-09989-6

Levinas, E. (1961). *Totality and infinity: An essay on exteriority* (Vol. 1). Springer Science & Business Media.

Lindsey, E. (1996). Health within illness: Experiences of chronically ill/disabled people. *Journal of Advanced Nursing, 24*(3), 465–472.

McGilchrist, I. (2009). *The master and his emissary: The divided brain and the making of the western world*. Yale University Press.

McGilchrist, I. (2011). *Can the divided brain tell us anything about the ultimate nature of reality*. Royal College of Psychiatrists.

McWhinney, I. (1997). *Textbook of family medicine*. Oxford University Press.

Merleau-Ponty, M. (1945). *Phénoménologie de la perception*. Gallimard. For the English translation: Merleau-Ponty, M. (1962). *Phenomenology of Perception* (C. Smith, Trans.). Routledge & Kegan Paul.

Merleau-Ponty, M. (2002). *The world of perception*. Routledge.

Mishler, E. (1984). *The discourse of medicine: Dialectics of medical interviews*. Ablex.

Mishler, E. (2005). Patient stories, narratives of resistance and the ethics of humane care: A la recherche du temps perdu. *Health, 9*(4), 431–451. https://doi.org/10.1177/1363459305056412

Norberg Boysen, G., Nyström, M., Christensson, L., Herlitz, J., & Wireklint Sundström, B. (2017). Trust in the early chain of healthcare: Lifeworld hermeneutics from the patient's perspective. *International Journal of Qualitative Studies on Health and Well-being, 12*(1), 1356674. https://doi.org/10.1080/17482631.2017.1356674

Pohlhaus, G., Jr. (2012). Relational knowing and epistemic injustice: Toward a theory of willful hermeneutical ignorance. *Hypatia, 27*(4), 715–735.

Pollard, C. (2015). What is the right thing to do: Use of a relational ethic framework to guide clinical decision-making. *International Journal of Caring Sciences, 8*(2), 362–368.

Reeve, J. (2010). Interpretive medicine: Supporting generalism in a changing primary care world. *Occasional Paper (Royal College of General Practitioners). 88*, 1–20.

Reeve, J. (2017). Unlocking the creative capacity of the self. In C. Dowrick (Ed.), *Person-centred primary care* (pp. 141–165). Routledge.

Russo, M. T. (2021). Ricoeur's hermeneutic arc and the "narrative turn" in the ethics of care. *Medicine, Health Care and Philosophy, 24*(3), 443–452.

Sandvik, H., Hetlevik, Ø., Blinkenberg, J., & Hunskaar, S. (2022). Continuity in general practice as predictor of mortality, acute hospitalisation, and use of out-of-hours care: A registry-based observational study in Norway. *British Journal of General Practice, 72*(715), e84–e90.

Savage, R., & Armstrong, D. (1990). Effect of a general practitioner's consulting style on patients' satisfaction: A controlled study. *British Medical Journal, 301*(6758), 968–970. https://doi.org/10.1136/bmj.301.6758.968

Schwartz, M., & Wiggins, O. (1985). Science, humanism, and the nature of medical practice: A phenomenological view. *Perspectives in Biology and Medicine, 28*(3), 331–361.

Shah, R., Ahluwalia, S., & Spicer, J. (2023). Relational care and epistemic injustice. *Primary Health Care Research & Development, 24*, e62. https://doi.org/10.1017/S1463423623000555

Shah, R., & Foell, J. (2024). *Fighting for the soul of general practice: The algorithm will see you now.* Intellect Books.

Spicer, J., Ahluwalia, S., & Shah, R. (2021). Moral flux in primary care: The effect of complexity. *Journal of Medical Ethics, 47*(2), 86–89 . https://doi.org/10.1136/medethics-2020-106149

Svenaeus, F. (2022). *The hermeneutics of medicine and the phenomenology of health: Steps towards a philosophy of medical practice* (Vol. 97). Springer.

Sweeney, K., Toy, L., & Cornwell, J. (2009). A patient's journey. *British Medical Journal, 339*, 511–551.

Sweeney, K. G., MacAuley, D., & Gray, D. P. (1998). Personal significance: The third dimension. *The Lancet, 351*(9096), 134–136.

Taylor, F. (1911). *The principles of scientific management.* Harper & Brothers.

Toombs, S. (1987). The meaning of illness: A phenomenological approach to the patient-physician relationship. *The Journal of Medicine and Philosophy, 12*(3), 219–240.

Wardrope, A., & Reuber, M. (2022). The hermeneutics of symptoms. *Medicine, Health Care and Philosophy, 25*(3), 395–412. https://doi.org/10.1007/s11019-022-10086-z

Whitehead, A. (1925). *Science and the modern world: Lowell lectures, 1925.* New American Library.

7 A hermeneutic approach to social injustice

Austin O'Carroll

There are people who reside on the shadowy margins of our society. They live there for a variety of reasons, including not having financial resources; not having a home; being addicted to alcohol or drugs; or coming from a foreign country. Patients who live on the margins have the worst health indices, having significantly shorter lifespans and spending more years of their shorter lives affected by disease (Baggett et al., 2010; Galea & Vlahov, 2002; Hwang et al., 2009; O'Reilly et al., 2015; Story, 2013).

We often describe these people being excluded from society and use the metaphor of 'barriers' to describe the multiple forms of exclusion (Figure 7.1). For example, we talk of barriers to education, barriers to healthcare, barriers to housing, etc. Barriers can be understood as being physical (e.g. stairs are a physical barrier for people using wheelchairs); administrative (e.g. forms in English are a barrier for people who are illiterate or do not speak English); attitudinal (stigmatising attitudes are some of the most invidious barriers); and finally, internalised barriers (e.g. if a person presumes they will be discriminated against if they attend a service, they will often decide not to attend, i.e. they have internalised the barrier).

In this chapter, we will explore a new concept, that of hermeneutic barriers in healthcare and how such barriers impact on the health of marginalised patients. A number of examples are proffered, demonstrating the existence and variety

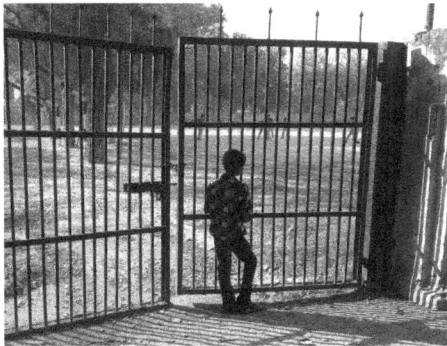

Figure 7.1 Marginalised Child (Banswalhemant, 2019).

DOI: 10.4324/9781003517665-7

of hermeneutic barriers, but there are many others. The objective is to create an awareness for practitioners working with patients from the margins of how hermeneutic barriers can be created on both sides of the clinician-patient relationship that result in such patients receiving sub-standard care. Having such an awareness can augment the ability of the practitioner to explore the assumptions and meanings adopted by individual marginalised patients, as outlined in the Four Domain Model of communication proposed by Shah et al. (2020). As they suggest, this would include exploring the patient's understanding of their illness experience and situation; the health professional reflecting on their own assumptions and biases; and lastly, identifying the external factors impacting on the consultation (e.g. the nature of homelessness/addiction). This should improve the health professional's ability to help patients overcome the hermeneutic barriers to accessing the healthcare they need.

In her book, *Epistemic Injustice: Power and Ethics of Unknowing*, Miranda Fricker describes her concept of hermeneutic injustice whereby those who have power in society control the creation of meaning:

> "It is obvious that certain material advantages will generate the envisaged epistemological advantage – if you have material power then you will tend to have an influence on those practices by which social meanings are generated." This control over meaning results in an unjust situation where "the powerful tend to have appropriate understanding of their experiences, ready to draw on as they make sense of their social experiences, whereas the powerless are more likely to find themselves having some social experiences through a glass darkly, with at best, ill-filling meanings to draw on in an effort to render them intelligible." She goes on to describe hermeneutic marginalisation. When 'there is unequal hermeneutic participation with respect to some significant area(s) of social experience, members of the disadvantaged group are hermeneutically marginalised. The notion of marginalisation is a moral-political one indicating subordination and exclusion from some practice that would have value for the participants.'
>
> (Fricker, 2007)

Hermeneutic barriers are a form of hermeneutic marginalisation/injustice. A hermeneutic barrier exists when there is a difference of sense making between members of the powerful majority and members of the marginalised group, resulting in those in the marginalised group having reduced access to the factors that promote health. One of the most important of these factors is the healthcare service.

These hermeneutic barriers can take two forms. The first form arises when the majority population makes sense of the behaviours of those from marginalised populations in a way that results in stigmatising and prejudicial beliefs and attitudes that, in turn, results in discriminatory behaviour towards members of the marginalised population. As those who work in the health services are members of the majority population, this discrimination can directly impact access to health services. The second form arises when the difference in sense making results in the creation of internalised barriers in members of the marginalised groups, resulting in them avoiding accessing health services. Importantly, the term is internalised, not internal, i.e. the barrier originates in the person's environment and is then internalised. So, for example, a person who has become a drug user may internalise the widespread societal attitude that people who use drugs are to blame for their poor health and are therefore not deserving of care; and so they may decide not to seek help for any of their health problems. They have internalised negative societal attitudes, resulting in an internalised barrier to accessing healthcare. Helping them overcome this internalised barrier may take the form of explaining to them that the research suggests most people who use drugs do so due to childhood experiences of trauma and/or poverty. Thus, it is not their individual fault but that of society for creating the conditions that create poverty/trauma. This can help them to create an alternative meaning for their drug using behaviour and so overcome their internalised barriers.

Let us start with the clinician and how their sense making of the world can create hermeneutic barriers. It has been argued that misunderstanding between two individuals that arises from perceiving different meanings inherent in an encounter can occur because of hastiness or prejudice. The latter can repeatedly and systematically recur, because if one has a prejudice, it will infuse every consultation that occurs with patients who are the object of that prejudice (Schleiermacher, 1998). When we discuss stigma, people often talk in terms of eradicating prejudice. However, eradicating prejudices implies that prejudice occurs fully at the conscious level and a decision to change one's thoughts can result in a deletion of the offending attitude. Gadamer (1989) argues differently, that our task is not to rid ourselves of biases and assumptions, but rather to become aware of them and recognise when they are negatively impacting on our relationships (Gadamer, 1989). This requires a constant reflection-in-action to identify when one's biases are acting in the moment so that one can take action to redress the impact of one's discriminatory behaviour.

Stephen and Joanne were two patients of mine who were rough sleeping in an inner-city park. They had been there several years. They refused to engage with most services and spent their days taking heroin, alcohol and crack cocaine. One winter Sunday, when all services were closed, their tent was blown down by a storm and they wandered the streets, wet and freezing. Eventually Stephen developed hypothermia, and they ended up in hospital, where he lost consciousness.

As the doctor and nurse were cutting off his clothes, the doctor turned to Joanne and said the condition they had got themselves into was disgraceful. When Stephen recovered and was discharged, both Joanne and Stephen swore they would never go to hospital again unless they were close to death as they did not want to face such shame-inducing situations. The doctor and possibly the nurse perceived that Stephen and Joanne had full agency over their decisions in life and that a decision to take drugs, alcohol and sleep rough was an autonomous one, made by two 'rational' human beings. As the 'rational' decision was such a bad one for their health and well-being, the doctor interpreted the decision as being disgraceful. Unfortunately, he did not take into account the huge impact of trauma and poverty on patients' behaviours and life choices. Malle (2004) provided a comprehensive and nuanced theory of attribution by considering not only how behaviour is explained, but also what behaviours are explained and why. Two types of explanations are reason explanations and causal history explanations. Reason explanations assume that the person is behaving according to their beliefs, desires and values. This is in contrast to causal history explanations that might imply reasons, but do not state them – such as the patient is 'non-compliant,' does not care, or does not want to listen. These explanations do not explicitly provide reasons based on beliefs, desires or values and are more likely to be employed in relation to marginalised groups (Malle, 2004).

Prejudice is in essence a hermeneutic barrier whereby people ascribe meanings to others' behaviours based on preconceived and simplistic stereotypes. To be fair, prejudices are more likely to surface in a stressful context, such as an over-busy Emergency Department. The sad thing is that most healthcare practitioners choose their career because they want to make a positive difference to other people's lives. The prejudice in this situation not only resulted in Stephen and Joanne developing internalised barriers to accessing healthcare, but also could be the source of moral injury for the doctor, who has not acted in accordance with the principles that brought him into medicine. Everyone has lost out. This is highlighted by what happened subsequently. A few months later, Stephen and Joanne entered a Safetynet (specialised service for homeless people) Mobile Health Unit, where they met a GP trainee. They were treated empathically and with respect while they had their chest infections treated. Of note, this doctor had been trained in trauma-Informed care. While they were there, the doctor persuaded them to attend a clinic that provided addiction treatment, where they started on opiate substitute treatment and were admitted to an alcohol detoxification programme. They were then housed and joined an educational programme. Joanne has since graduated from Ireland's top university and is starting a Master's programme.

Another common example of prejudice resulting in a hermeneutic barrier is shown by the way in which practitioners react when patients do not comply with treatment. Thirsk et al. (2014) described the reactions of nurses encountering patients who failed to listen to medical advice about treatment for their kidney disease. A commonly ascribed meaning was that the person had made a personal choice, perhaps because of their character; and therefore, very little could be done to help them. In contrast, other nurses viewed the context within which the person made the choice not to have treatment, e.g. were they stressed by the hospital environment; were they a single parent with children to look after; did they have a substance misuse issue? These nurses were more likely to address the barriers that prevented the person accepting the treatment. As the authors noted, 'how nurses explain or attribute a patient's behaviour influences their subsequent actions' and it was evident 'that the interventions following an attribution of behaviour to non-compliance would differ significantly from the interventions following an attribution of behaviour to varied, understandable circumstances' (Thirsk et al., 2014). The labelling of patients as non-compliant has been critiqued in the nursing literature (Russell et al., 2003; Wright & Marie, 1992). It has been emphasised that nurses need to consider a social model of health where 'health and illness are features of the complex and interactive system commonly referred to as life' (Russell et al., 2003).

It is not just individuals who make assumptions about how people make sense of and identify value in their lives. Systems also do this. Take, for example, hospital outpatients. If one maintains the view that people are rational decision makers and a failure to keep an appointment is an autonomous choice, then one fails to see the hugely damaging health inequity created by an appointment system that obviously does not work. Hospitals have for years been sending appointments by post to people experiencing homelessness, the stupidest thing I have come across in my career as a doctor. Every morning in my clinic, I open letter after letter telling me that a patient has failed to attend their outpatient appointment and that they have therefore been discharged. There is the obvious issue that people experiencing homelessness will not receive appointment letters, as they have no permanent address. However, that is not the only issue. Those of us who don't live on the margins of society tend to have regular lives where we know from day to day where we will be. We keep diaries to ensure we will not miss important meetings or appointments. We tend to value our lives – our families, our homes, our jobs, our holidays, our prospects and our children's prospects – and we want to remain in good health to continue enjoying all these rich aspects of our lives. People experiencing homelessness have chaotic lives where they do not know what they will be doing from day to day, nor where they will be staying from week to week. They do not keep diaries. They are not as happy with their lives, which are often littered with trauma and failures, resulting in low self-esteem and shame. So, they do not value their health in the same way as those of us who have a more certain place in society. As a result, they are less likely to keep hospital appointments.

When the new hepatitis C treatments emerged, which had 95–99% success rates in clearing the disease, I referred 40 of my patients to the local hepatology service. 23 missed their first appointment, seven their second and only two completed treatment. Stupid patients or stupid medicine? We decided stupid medicine. We did not see people experiencing homelessness as rational decision makers who had decided not to take care of their health. We saw the appointment system as one designed for the needs of the housed majority, that was poorly suited to the needs of the homeless. So, we came up with a different model for our patients. We worked with our local infectious disease service, so that instead of the patient having to attend seven hospital appointments, the majority of assessments and interventions now take place in our primary care clinic, with only one compulsory hospital appointment. We recruited a peer support worker, Bernard West, who had himself been homeless and had previously been infected with hepatitis C, to help us ensure people complied with the programme. All 40 people were treated and many more have been treated since. This model works. We have also developed models where secondary care is delivered in homeless services for diabetes, chronic obstructive pulmonary disease, epilepsy and deep vein thrombosis; and we are developing a photo-based referral system for dermatology.

However, it is not just at the systemic level that how we make meaning acts as a barrier for marginalised groups. Hermeneutic barriers are also created by how we organise our medical epistemology. Take, for example, how we respond to young people who are at risk of taking their own lives, based on the medical epistemology of suicidality.

At the start of clinic that morning, Thomas, the clinic manager, told me two of our clients had died that week. One had died from an overdose. The other, an older drinker, had been found dead on the street. Piotr was my sixth client that morning. He came with a young female keyworker. He had an angry red, swollen abscess in his groin, where he had been injecting for the last six weeks. His keyworker told me he had overdosed twice in the previous two weeks. I listened to his story, which was brief. I asked questions, including checking whether he had intended on committing suicide. He replied he was not trying to take his own life, but he added, as an afterthought, that he did not care whether he lived or died. The infection was bad. His hold on life was tenuous. I told him he needed to go to hospital, both to get the abscess drained and also to have a psychiatric review. He refused: 'Just give me some antibiotics. I will be fine.' I pleaded with him. I cajoled him. I tried to bribe him with a promise of a benzodiazepine maintenance course and nutritional drinks (both of which he needed anyway) if he would go in. All to no avail. I told him I was worried about him, I cared about him and I did not want him to die. We agreed that I would provide the antibiotics and nutritional drinks, sign him up for opiate substitute treatment and he would come back to us the following day. His keyworker said she would chase him down to make sure he attended. I discussed his case with the psychiatrist on call to see if he would warrant a compulsory admission. The psychiatrist's opinion was that though Piotr did not care whether he lived or died, he was not intending to kill himself and further as he was under the influence of drugs, this implied that he had no active intention to die. Therefore, he did not warrant psychiatric compulsory admission.

Piotr and I ascribe different meanings to our lives. My life is filled with 'meaning,' in that I see myself as part of a family, as a father to children, as a son to my mother and brother to my siblings, as a person with an array of friends who care for me, as a valued colleague at work, as a person who enjoys life and contributes to the happiness of others. Piotr does not see these meanings in his life and so life has less meaning for him.

More importantly, the psychiatrist and I ascribe different meanings to our store of clinical knowledge and our understanding of our roles as doctors to this patient. I see little difference between taking actions that will likely kill oneself because of an active intention to take one's life; compared to taking actions that are likely to result in death because one does not care whether one lives or dies. However, within medical epistemology, seeking to die intentionally is perceived as a mental illness warranting compulsory admission, whereas caring so little for your life that you take high risks with it is not identified as a mental illness. Unfortunately, these presumptions can end up as being classist, because taking high risks due to addiction and homelessness mainly affects people from impoverished communities, whereas suicidality affects all strata of society. It behoves practitioners, when adopting a hermeneutic approach, to also critically evaluate the biases and assumptions inherent in our clinical knowledge and practice.

Now let us explore examples of how patients making meaning of their worlds can result in internalised hermeneutic barriers to health and healthcare. We make sense of our world by interacting with and observing others. Thus, most of us who are not socially disadvantaged presume we will live a long life, surrounded as we are by people surviving into their 80s or 90s. As we know we are likely to live such a long time, we take care of our heath by attending screening programmes, accessing healthcare when we have potentially worrying symptoms and following clinical advice about how to remain healthy and maximise our lifespan.

However, imagine if instead, we lived in a community where many people die in their twenties and thirties and very few people live past 60 years old. Imagine that in this community, one in three has a serious life-threatening infection, one in two suffers from depression, one in three attempts suicide at some stage in their lives, with one in five having made this attempt in the previous six months (O'Reilly et al., 2015). It has been recognised that one of the reasons homeless people do not attend health services is based on their belief that they will not live very long, so there is little point in taking care of their health. This assumption is realistic, when one understands the experiences of premature death that pervade the everyday lives of homeless people. If health professionals consider the actions of homeless people not taking care of their health as being the autonomous choices of rational humans who have actively chosen drugs over health, then they will be unable to address this internalised barrier. When I encounter an internalised barrier, I emphasise repeatedly the life potential that exists for my patient and how as clinicians, we can help them to live a long life if they will help us manage their health.

Another example of an internalised barrier relates to how homeless people and the housed majority have different understandings of space; and the way in which this can result in exclusion. It is recognised that homeless people have poor attendance rates in primary care and often leave emergency department or outpatient waiting rooms before they are seen. It is often presumed that this is due to them having other, competing priorities to attend to, e.g. obtaining illicit drugs or alcohol; seeking food; obtaining accommodation (Cheallaigh et al., 2017). The possibility that the waiting room space itself is the barrier, and the meaning homeless people attach to waiting rooms is not considered.

They say the plastic seats in Fast Food joints are designed to become uncomfortable after 20 minutes, just enough time to finish one's fast meal. The seat I sat in in the waiting room of the Emergency Department had a similar design, but I, along with the 20–30 other people there had sat in these seats for over four hours. There was a hum of conversation as people waited their long turn to be called up by the nurse to triage or to enter the clinical area. Some people drank machine-produced tea or coffee and munched on machine-produced snacks. I sensed everyone was watching where they were in the queue and scanning to ensure they were not overlooked.

Suddenly, the back door opened. An unkempt woman in a blue tracksuit, hair in a pony-tail, entered carrying a bottle of vodka. She scanned the room aggressively, as if daring anyone to look back at her. The room went silent. 'Are you coming in or not,' she said loudly in an inner-city Dublin accent. An unshaven man, with poorly cut hair, wearing a hoodie and tracksuit bottoms followed her in, cigarette in his hand. I, and I suspect the rest of the people in the room, presumed they were both homeless and/or drug users and/ or alcoholics.

They walked slowly, alongside the wall, around the room talking loudly, their conversation peppered with fucks and other swear words. They went into the toilet. Though no one spoke, the atmosphere in the room seemed to relax. That is, until they came out. They slank along the wall, again talking loudly and antagonistically and then left. After 30 seconds, people started to slowly wind back into conversation and the tension eased.

I followed our two friends and found them sitting on the back steps of the old entrance door to the Emergency Department, with four other equally unkempt people, two with bottles of vodka in their hands and all with cigarettes. However, the atmosphere was different. They greeted me. They were chatting, cracking jokes, bantering. There was plenty of swearing but it was fucking for fun, not for fear. It reminded me of being in the kitchen at a 1980s house party, where everyone knew the real fun and craic was to be found. This was the first time I became aware of how both homeless and housed people attach different meanings to space. The waiting room space was the territory of the housed, who felt at ease there; while the concrete steps were the territory of the unhoused, drinkers and drug users. Invasion of each other's space caused tension and fear for both parties. The first meaning we apply to space is 'mine' or 'not mine.' The second is 'safe' or 'not safe,' where safety can be interpreted in terms of physical safety from assault or injury or emotional safety from being made to feel inferior or unwanted. People experiencing homelessness often feel conspicuous and shamed in hospital or waiting rooms, where they suspect that other people are looking down on them (O'Carroll & Wainwright, 2019). It is understood as not being their space, as a space that is not safe and will cause painful emotions. Thus, they avoid such spaces even if it means losing out on access to the healthcare that lies on the other side of the doors bordering the space. Thus, space itself can be a hermeneutic barrier.

Specialised services are services for marginalised groups that are specifically designed to meet their needs. They are usually located in spaces that people experiencing homelessness feel comfortable in. For example, in Dublin, there is a GP/ Nurse run clinic supported by a translator, located in the Capuchin centre – a food hall serving meals to over 600 homeless and migrant people daily. The contrast between the waiting area in this centre and that in the Emergency Department is stark. People experiencing homelessness come in and queue for their meal, saying hello to each other, seeking out familiar faces and shaking hands. This includes both older people who look like they have alcohol problems or mental health problems and younger people who look like they have drug problems. It is almost carnival like. At one end of the hall is a small area where people sit on benches outside two surgery rooms. They are queuing for the nurse or doctor; and like the others in the hall they are talking and laughing with each other. This is their space, where they feel safe and comfortable to wait for the healthcare on the other side of the door.

I encountered another interesting example of a space-related hermeneutic barrier to healthcare when working on the streets. John was a rough sleeper who slept in the same inner-city park for over nine years. It took me a while to develop a relationship with him. When I visited him, he would interview me like a barrister, weigh up whether he would like to avail of my services or not, and if not, would dismiss me with an imperious wave of his hand. This was his consulting space, not mine. We eventually persuaded him to enter a long-term hostel for homeless people. When I visited him in the hostel, he acted more deferentially and seemed more anxious in my company. I surmised that being outside his space made him feel less safe and comfortable and less able to exercise his autonomy in making decisions about his health. The meaning he applied to space resulted in a flipping of power dynamics once he was housed.

In all the examples so far, I have concentrated on examples of barriers to accessing healthcare. In this last example, I want to describe a different hermeneutic barrier to health: people who complete higher education live longer and healthier lives (Zajacova & Lawrence, 2018).

Kathleen was 16 years old. She attended our practice regularly, either with her mother, a 45-year-old woman who had a severe alcohol problem and chronic obstructive pulmonary disease or with her mother and her 12 year old brother who had a diagnosis of attention deficit disorder and significant behavioural issues at school. She would tell the GP what was wrong with her mother or brother, help her mother and brother answer the doctor's questions and then listen closely as they outlined the proposed treatment. I met her on a few occasions doing the shopping for the family. She would always say hello and smile at me.

One day she came with her mother who beamed with pride. 'Guess what?', she said. 'Kathleen got nine honours in the Junior Certificate.' 'Wow!' I replied. This was impressive. Kathleen was clearly one super smart girl if she could manage her mother and brother and still get nine honours. I congratulated her and enthusiastically asked if she would consider going to college after she had completed school and done her Leaving Certificate, two years hence. She looked at me quizzically. 'Do the Leaving Cert' she said bemused. 'I am leaving school next week.' She was going to become a hairdresser. I tried to dissuade her. I got her to see a counsellor. I got her to see a schools' officer. She still left. Two years later, she was a single mother. She was delighted to have a child aged 18 years old. Four years after this, she presented frequently, seeking benzodiazepines for anxiety. When I was her age, I did not just hope to go to college, I (probably arrogantly) presumed it. When I was her age, I did not envision having children till I was in my late twenties at the earliest. For her, having an education offered no value, whereas having children provided her with a caring role that she had previously adopted with her mother and brother. However, the result is that her chances of having a long and healthy life have been significantly reduced. This is a hermeneutic barrier to health. The clinician in this situation has a dilemma: should she challenge Kathleen to try to persuade her to stay in school or should she accept it is her choice to leave? There is no clear answer, but I believe that Kathleen did not have a clear choice, because even the notion of going to college had not occurred to her. I have challenged other people in similar situations, and some have gone to college which has transformed their lives. There is a constant balance to be struck between challenge and respect.

So, what is the pragmatic value of the concept of a hermeneutic barrier? Fricker has described hermeneutic justice and what she calls a virtuous hearer.

A virtuous hearer is someone who seeks to understand the meaning that the narrator attaches to their experiences. The virtuous hearer seeks to avoid imposing their own preformed understandings of the issues being discussed in the narrator's story and rather seeks to understand the meaning held by the narrator. This requires self-reflection and an awareness of one's internalised prejudices (Fricker, 2007). Thus, for example, a practitioner who listens to an account of a person who describes their use of heroin can either impose their own meaning – that such behaviour reflects a self-indulgent lack of moral fibre; or they can choose to hear how the person takes drugs as a form of self-medication, to ease the pain of their own past and present traumatic experiences. This approach is in line with Shah et al. (2020), who propose that practitioners should continuously reflect on spoken and unspoken meanings during clinical encounters, in order to help patients navigate their illness. For marginalised populations, such a navigation may include opening up the hermeneutic barriers that exist on the path to healthcare and health.

Practitioners must prevent hermeneutic barriers impeding access for those patients who most need healthcare. This involves firstly, preventing the construction of hermeneutic barriers; secondly, identifying the existence of hermeneutic barriers; and lastly, taking action to destroy or diminish those barriers.

1   Preventing the construction of hermeneutic barriers.

   a   Be a virtuous hearer and seek to understand the actual meaning of what your patients are saying. This requires an understanding of their background coupled with knowledge of how a traumatic background can warp communication. Thus, a patient who tells you they do not care about their untreated hepatitis C, may actually be saying 'I am too caught in up in drug addiction, which I use to calm the emotions arising from my past trauma to have time to focus on getting my hepatitis treated'; or they may be saying 'I think I am going to die young anyway, so treating this is of no value to me.' If it is the former, then getting them onto treatment for their addiction is the primary aim before getting them to address their hepatitis C. If it is the latter, the solution lies in being there for them and outlining a future where they can live a fruitful and fulfilling life.

   b   Constantly reflect on your words and actions. Reflection-on-action is where you engage in reflective activities after the event, e.g. through writing or through group support (e.g. Balint groups). Reflection-in-action is reflection during the encounter. One develops the ability to reflect in action by reflecting on action.

   c   Remember the Hermeneutic Window when working with people experiencing homelessness and provide holistic care that combines evidence based practice with creation of meaning and narrative humility

2   Identifying hermeneutic barriers

   a   Reflect on your own words and actions as above.

   b   Reflect on the administrative and communicative practices and potential stigma within your workplace. Access training in trauma-informed care. Identify barriers to care in your own workplace.

3 Taking action to destroy or diminish hermeneutic barriers

    a Constantly survey your own actions and words and apologise when you see they have unintentionally caused barriers or offence. Learn to change your practice when you have identified actions that cause barriers.

    b Engage your team to come up with solutions to the barriers that are identified within your workplace.

    c Involve patients in solutions. This can involve using surveys, focus groups and employing peer workers. We now have several peer workers working in our service who provide invaluable feedback to us on how we can improve access.

The biomedical model has become the paramount, dominant paradigm for addressing the health needs of our patients. The biomedical model seeks to cast practitioners as dispassionate scientists making rational, scientific assessments of their patients' health and spewing out evidence based treatments or referrals in accordance with guidelines. Such a reductionist approach ignores the reality of the lived experience of our patients, particularly marginalised populations.

I met her standing outside the hospital in her dressing gown and pyjamas, a cigarette in her hands. She smiled and waved at me. 'What are you doing in hospital,' I asked. 'Me? Breathing!' she replied. 'This COPD is getting to me.' I looked at her cigarette with a quizzical look on my face. 'I know, I know,' she laughed. 'But you can't expect me to give up smoking. Look at all I have given up already. I am doing so much better.' She was right. She had given up heroin. She had given up benzodiazepines. She had given up alcohol. She had given up crack cocaine. She had given up methadone, though she kept tight hold of her regular diazepam prescription. And she had improved. She had got treatment for her hepatitis C. She had put on weight. She had started on inhalers for her COPD. I remember a conversation I had with her about giving up cigarettes in the recent past, pressing for that last change. 'You are asking too much,' she had said. 'These little fags are the only thing I have in my life beside me kids, and they are in care.' I warned of the effect on her lungs, but she said she would be ok. She had come through too much to give up now.

References

Baggett, T., O'Connell, J., Singer, D., & Rigotti, N. (2010). The unmet health care needs of homeless adults: A national study. *American Journal of Public Health*, *100*(7), 1326–1333.

Banswalhemant. (2019). *Marginalised child in Delhi*. (Photo) Wikimedia Commons. https://commons.wikimedia.org/wiki/File:Marginalised_child_in_Delhi.jpg

Cheallaigh, C., Cullivan, S., Sears, J., Lawlee, A., Browne, J., Kieran, J., Segurado, R., O'Carroll, A., O'Reilly, F., & Creagh, D. (2017). Usage of unscheduled hospital care by homeless individuals in Dublin, Ireland: A cross-sectional study. *BMJ Open*, *7*(11), e016420.

Fricker, M. (2007). *Epistemic injustice: Power and the ethics of knowing*. Oxford University Press.

Gadamer, H.- G. (1989). *Truth and method*. A&C Black.

Galea, S., & Vlahov, D. (2002). Social determinants and the health of drug users: Socioeconomic status, homelessness, and incarceration. *Public Health Reports*, *117*(Suppl 1), S135.

Hwang, S., Wilkins, R., Tjepkema, M., O'Campo, P., & Dunn, J. (2009). Mortality among residents of shelters, rooming houses, and hotels in Canada: 11 year follow-up study. *British Medical Journal*, *339*, b4036. https://doi.org/10.1136/bmj.b4036

Malle, B. (2004). *How the mind explains behavior: Folk explanations, meaning, and social interaction*. MIT press.

O'Carroll, A., & Wainwright, D. (2019). Making sense of street chaos: An ethnographic exploration of homeless people's health service utilization. *International Journal for Equity in Health*, *18*, 1–22.

O'Reilly, F., Barror, S., Hannigan, A., Scriver, S., Ruane, L., MacFarlane, A., & O'Carroll, A. (2015). *Homelessness: An unhealthy state. health status, risk behaviours and service utilisation among homeless people in two Irish cities* (pp. 0–96). Dublin: The Partnership for Health Equity.

Russell, S., Daly, J., Hughes, E., & Hoog, C. (2003). Nurses and 'difficult' patients: Negotiating non-compliance. *Journal of advanced nursing*, *43*(3), 281–287.

Schleiermacher, F. (1998). *Hermeneutics and criticism and other writings* (A. Bowie, Trans.). Cambridge University Press.

Shah, R., Clarke, R., Ahluwalia, S., & Launer, J. (2020). Finding meaning in the consultation: Introducing the hermeneutic window. *British Journal of General Practice*, *70*(699), 502–503.

Story, A. (2013). Slopes and cliffs in health inequalities: Comparative morbidity of housed and homeless people. *The Lancet*, *382*, S93.

Thirsk, L., Moore, S., & Keyko, K. (2014). Influences on clinical reasoning in family and psychosocial interventions in nursing practice with patients and their families living with chronic kidney disease. *Journal of Advanced Nursing*, *70*(9), 2117–2127.

Wright, L., & Marie, A. (1992). The non-existence of non-compliant families: The influence of Humberto Maturana. *Journal of Advanced Nursing*, *17*(8), 913–917.

Zajacova, A., & Lawrence, E. (2018). The relationship between education and health: Reducing disparities through a contextual approach. *Annual Review of Public Health*, *39*(1), 273–289.

8 The human element in the age of AI

Balancing technology and meaning in medicine

Marcus Lewis, Sylvie Delacroix,
David Fraile Navarro and Richard Lehman

A short history of technology in primary care

A major problem with discussing artificial intelligence (AI) is the differing conceptions people have of what it is and isn't. Here one of us (RL) describes how the use of 'Health Informatics' affected his own practice during his years as a GP in a small town in middle England between 1979 and 2015. This gives a picture of how 'old AI,' a particularly limited and often botched implementation of health informatics, crept into the consulting room and came to dominate it. It was a clumsy little elephant which grew and grew, pushing itself between doctor and patient and often trampling on the relationship between them. Not only they grew apart, but more often it left doctors burned out (Adler-Milstein et al., 2020) especially as they must devote the sacred and scarce consultation time to fill mostly useless forms in a dystopian manner. Although this chapter carries a great warning, we rest optimistic about current and future usage of AIs, and particularly what has come to be known as Generative AI (GenAI). Later in this chapter, we make some suggestions about how it might mature into a powerful gentle friend who never forgets.

In 1979, I came as a young GP to a small practice in Banbury which had been set up by an early enthusiast for computing in general practice. The actual computer was nowhere to be seen. It occupied a large room in Oxford and had to be fed (at night, for reasons of telephone capacity) using reams of special green paper with holes down the sides. I knew in a vague way that computers were going to shape the future, so I decided to go along to a meeting of the Oxfordshire GP computer group who were jointly feeding the machine. It did not take me long to realise that I was in no position to understand what they were talking about or join their effort. It seemed to me that it would take decades before their systems would be anything more than a system of laboriously collecting basic epidemiological data.

That was a common mistake, of course. For people not engaged in the field, digital technology seems at every point to promise more than it can deliver. But in the next 15 years, it would deliver a world wide web, mobile phones, video game consoles and word processors in millions of households, and computers in every consulting room. And then things began to calm down somewhat, as we came to terms with the enormity of what had happened.

DOI: 10.4324/9781003517665-8

Small town English general practice at the end of the 1970s was conservative with both cases of the letter C. There were still traces of the world described in George Eliot's *Middlemarch* (published 1871–1872 and set around 1830). New-comers were not entirely welcome as they disturbed the balance of payments and threatened the stability of various arcane arrangements to do with capitation bound-aries, nursing homes, police work, pharmacy ownership and other long-held perks. None of this interested me so much as developing a practice which was as patient friendly as possible. I was not yet 30 and a little naïve. I knew I had a lot to learn.

Our practice was located very close to the local small general hospital and if patients were admitted, we wandered in by day or night and talked to the consult-ants looking after them. This seemed a perfectly normal way of learning medicine and keeping touch with patients. It never occurred to us to think of this in terms of trust-building or continuity of care: we simply took these for granted. Notes were written by hand for the guidance of ourselves and our immediate colleagues. Meanwhile, in the world of GP training, various local doctors were pioneering the teaching of communication skills and consultation analysis using early video. In the country at large, the Conservatives with a capital C were making noises that threatened the stability of the NHS, but in our little pocket we were going through a mini golden age.

Then came the disruptive technology. To me, it seemed much too disruptive from the start. Its only obvious advantage was that it made repeat prescribing eas-ier. For that, you had to mount a heavy cathode ray monitor and a keyboard on your desk. As I believed in using the smallest possible desk to avoid any barrier between myself and patients, this already seemed wrong. And the late morning ritual of writing out repeat prescriptions had been a great opportunity to sit with colleagues drinking coffee and exchanging ideas and gossip. A Luddite before the age of 40, I held out against computers in the surgery for as long as possible. But late in 1989 I went off for a sabbatical in New Zealand and my partners took the opportunity of getting them set up in my absence. It was inevitable anyway. Before long, no GP practice could draw payments without using these machines to claim items of service and satisfy mandatory auditing requirements.

This was hardly AI. In fact, it was artificial dumbing down. We took on extra staff to feed the machine, and to tell us what we were doing wrong: not as doctors, of course, but as machine feeders. The machine needed data. Some of this was provided by staff laboriously transcribing laboratory reports and physical measure-ments from non-compatible hospital systems. Some of it was provided as diagnos-tic codes after each consultation. And so, over the next decades up to the present, the focus of general practice moved from unmediated conversation with patients towards a constant anxiety about diagnostic test results, data input, and arriving at a diagnostic code for each encounter.

Still, you could ask, what has this to do with *real* AI? Nothing and everything. Nothing, in the sense that these machines were unintelligent in the extreme. You had to do all their thinking for them, and this was very boring and time-consuming. Everything, in the sense that you were building up a huge data set that more sophis-ticated 'intelligent' systems could later be trained to 'think' with.

The clinical coding side of medical computing struck me as outright dangerous from the start. We fumbled badly with those early Read Codes and quickly
found a tiny subset that covered our pressing need to enter a number and call the
next patient. We scanned hospital letters and highlighted diagnoses for our clerical staff to add to the tally for each patient. A label once attached is difficult to
remove. And so the grand datasets, which the NHS is now so proud of, contain
every conjectural diagnosis or convenient shortcut made by rushed doctors over
the last 30 years. It is a lucky patient indeed who does not have some garbage in
their record which could mislead other health professionals or might affect their
chance of insurance.

But on the positive side, this period – the early 1990s – also saw the birth of
'evidence based medicine' (EBM), which was critically enabled by new ways of
accessing evidence and analysing it by computational methods. I bridled a bit at the
term, as if we had been practising without evidence until taught to do so by certain
Canadians. But actually I warmed to those (mainly) Canadians because they promised a better kind of science to underlie patient care.

The rest of my working life has been spent largely in various kinds of dialogue
with EBM and meaning in medicine. The relationship between the way that medical evidence is conceptualised, tested and expressed is largely governed by aca-
demics, journals and the medical-industrial complex. It often bears little relation
to what patients seek help for, and in my view it misclassifies almost every aspect
of what medicine should really be about. These vitally important questions are
discussed elsewhere in this book. For the purposes of this chapter, I will simply
round off my personal story as a working GP as it relates to the arrival 'pre-AI' as
the consulting room elephant.

As the 1990s progressed, our clunky machines became increasingly able to
relay knowledge to us, rather than simply demand our input. Almost overnight, the
world wide web (or internet, as we now usually call it) enabled us to communicate
instantly over any distance, great or small. Electronic mail was the most obvious
use, but it was equally exciting to be able to look things up instantly that previously took hours of searching in libraries. This was the great enabler of evidence
based medicine at the bedside, as David Sackett taught it, using a huge trolley of
machinery. But only a few of the patients I saw were actually in bed. So it was for-
tunate that trolleys rapidly became redundant and we were soon able to do the same
using personal computers in our homely consulting rooms, and eventually mobile
devices in patients' homes.

At the same time, EBM enthusiasts were getting very keen on the new possibilities our machines provided for disseminating up to date summaries of evidence.
A whole new industry of systematic reviewing and guideline production sprang
up with surprising speed, so that by the end of the decade, the NHS already had a
central body which used rigorous literature reviews to decide on the effectiveness
of every new intervention – the National Institute for Health and Care Excellence
(NICE). These were heady days of good intentions. Our shelves filled with bulky
printed NICE guidelines, until they spilled over and threatened to injure toddlers
playing on the floor nearby.

But was the digital world becoming more intelligent? Hardly, but it was imping-ing more and more on the use and focus of our own intelligence. And when guide-lines became instantiated into a system of payment for 'quality' in clinical practice, the computer took an increasingly intrusive and sinister aspect. Hardly any con-sultations could be done without the appearance of a 'QOF prompt' (Quality and Outcomes Framework) reminding us that the practice might lose financially if we did not raise some issue or perform some action quite unrelated to what the patient had come about. To the visual distraction was added a distraction of priorities and trust. It was impossible for patients not to notice. This was the situation when I left my practice in 2010. I continued to undertake out-of-hours and locum work for another few years. Nothing I have read or heard makes me think the situation has changed for the better. Yet.

What is Generative AI?

GenAI holds both immense promise and potential challenges for the future of medicine. Given its rapid development, current GenAI models, trained on vast amounts of medical information, demonstrate a remarkable familiarity with medi-cal language and concepts. While these models don't possess genuine expertise or reason in the same way a human doctor does, their ability to generate fluent and accurate medical text is rapidly improving. These tools have moved from provid-ing entertaining but often erroneous answers into being able to answer complex medical questions and medical exam questions with remarkable accuracy (Saab et al., 2024). In the future, they may be able to sift through millions of patient records, identifying subtle patterns and predicting potential, personalised health risks. Moreover, GenAI can translate complex medical jargon into clear, concise language, making information accessible to all. We will explore how this technol-ogy could go even further, acting as a bridge between doctor and patient to facili-tate, rather than diminish, communication and understanding.

But how does this seemingly intelligent technology actually work? At its core, GenAI is powered by sophisticated 'neural' machine learning algorithms called large language models (LLMs). These language models are trained on vast amounts of human text, encompassing both medical and general knowledge, not to store information directly, but to learn the statistical relationships between words and concepts. In this learning process, they are trained to 'predict the next word,' but contrary to popular belief, by doing it, these 'stochastic parrots' (Bender et al., 2021) can learn true relationships between symptoms, diagnoses, treatments, and even the subtle patterns of language that clinicians use to describe their patients' experiences. This allows them not only to produce medical-grade summaries and clinical letters, but also to predict likely outcomes and identify course of actions, suggests tests or treatments and identify subtle connections and diagnostic options, even simulating the reasoning processes of human experts.

However, unlike the rigid, rule-based systems of the past, GenAI can adapt and evolve. It can use its vast knowledge base to craft language that is nuanced, context-aware, and strikingly similar to human expression. For instance, it can take a dense research paper filled with technical terms and create a concise summary that a patient (or a time-pressed doctor) could easily understand and action. It can even draft a personalised letter to a patient explaining a new diagnosis in a way that is both informative and compassionate.

This capacity for generating sophisticated and adaptable language opens up a world of possibilities in healthcare. Imagine a chatbot that can answer patients' basic health questions, providing reliable information and guidance outside of traditional clinic hours. Or a tool that can analyse a patient's medical history and generate a personalised list of potential health risks, empowering patients to take a more proactive role in their own care. Going even further, these tools could act as a liaison between patients and doctors allowing them to understand each other better.

Yet, as we navigate these possibilities, we should also consider the implications of a technology that can mimic human communication. Might relying too heavily on such a technology alter the delicate balance of understanding between doctor and patient? Could it inadvertently obscure the nuances of individual experience, the unspoken fears and hopes that shape a patient's understanding of illness? Does the use of this advanced form of automation and reasoning aid, carry the risk to 'downgrade' the clinical experience? Or will it lead to 'deskilling' of health professionals? These are questions worth pondering as we explore how this powerful technology might reshape the art of medicine.

What can be done using GenAI now and in the future?

GenAI is rapidly changing the landscape of medicine, with its influence extending from the mundane tasks of documentation to the complex challenges of diagnosis. While much attention focuses on the potential for AI to revolutionise how we diagnose diseases, a quieter revolution is already underway in the consulting room itself. AI scribes, listening in on consultations and automatically generating notes, are becoming increasingly commonplace in primary care. This integration of GenAI into clinical workflows is further exemplified by systems like the Madrid healthcare system, which has incorporated a custom version of ChatGPT into its electronic health records to assist clinicians with diagnosing rare diseases (Microsoft Prensa, 2023).

This apparent leap forward, however, is not without its complexities. While AI-assisted diagnosis offers the promise of increased accuracy, efficiency, and access to specialised knowledge, it also raises concerns about the potential for unintended consequences. Decades ago, Ivan Illich, in his seminal work *Medical Nemesis* (Illich, 1975), offered a prescient warning about the medicalisation of life: the tendency to view every human experience through a medical lens. He argued that this trend can lead to a loss of autonomy, an over-reliance on experts, and a diminishing of our capacity for self-care. Could GenAI, in its pursuit of diagnostic precision, exacerbate this trend, shifting power away from individuals and towards technology? Furthermore, the algorithm's voice, always ready with a diagnosis, risks overshadowing the patient's own narrative, potentially promoting a bias towards action rather than watchful waiting.

A doctor, accustomed to guiding patients through the uncertainties of diagnosis, might find themselves facing a new challenge: a patient who arrives with a smartphone printout confidently proclaiming an AI-generated diagnosis. This scenario echoes the familiar challenge posed by readily available online medical information, often referred to as 'Dr. Google.' However, unlike the varied and often easily interpretable results from a Google search, GenAI presents a distinct set of challenges, often providing definitive assessments without clear sourcing or references, delivered in an 'oracular' format that can be difficult for both patients and clinicians to decipher. This lack of transparency, coupled with the potential for AI hallucination (Pal & Sankarasubbu, 2024), undermines shared decision-making and a truly patient-centred approach to care. The patient, having meticulously inputted their symptoms, medical history, and even genetic information into the algorithm, now sits expectantly, awaiting the doctor's confirmation. In this scenario, the doctor's function is redefined, potentially shifting from primary interpreter of the patient's experience to a verifier of the AI's assessment. How does this reframing of the clinical encounter impact the doctor's ability to be a careful listener, to understand the nuances of the patient's story, and to address the 'why' behind their suffering?

The hermeneutic lens compels us to consider these questions. Hermeneutics, the art of understanding and interpretation, reminds us that medicine is not merely a matter of matching symptoms to diagnoses but of engaging with the unique story of each patient. The doctor-patient encounter is a delicate dance, a space where meaning is co-created through dialogue, empathy, and a shared understanding of the patient's world and journey. Figure 8.1 shows a dialogue between two people – in this case the philosophers Aristotle and Plato – both of whose perspectives are crucial to the emergence of a new meaning. The patient's narratives, their hopes, fears, values and beliefs, are not simply data to be fed into an algorithm; these are the very fabric of their illness experience.

However, we must acknowledge that achieving this ideal of shared meaning making can be challenging in today's healthcare environment. Strained resources, time pressures, and a growing emphasis on efficiency can often hinder the development

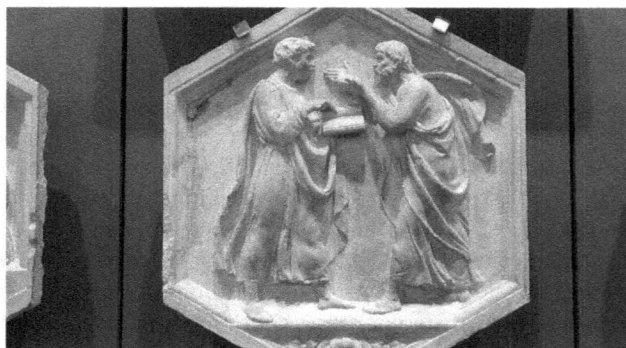

Figure 8.1 Meaning is Co-created: Relief Sculpture of Discourse/Dialectic between Plato and Aristotle (Hacklai, 2019).

of deep connections and truly patient-centred care. Despite these obstacles, the hermeneutic perspective provides a valuable framework for understanding the importance of narrative, empathy, and shared decision-making in the pursuit of healing.

GenAI, for all its potential, further risks disruption of this delicate process. In its quest for immediateness and diagnostic certainty, it could prioritise a standardised, data-driven approach over the messy, ambiguous realities of the human condition, encompassing both challenges and opportunities for healing. AI's strength in processing large datasets and identifying patterns could exacerbate the existing trend in medical practice towards normative inquiry – a symptom-focused approach that seeks to quickly categorise patients into predefined diagnostic boxes – and further distance it from the patient's unique story. This could lead to an even more fragmented and depersonalised approach to patient care. The patient, instead of being seen as a complex individual with a unique story to tell, might become reduced to a set of data points, their narrative overshadowed by the algorithm's pronouncements.

Therefore, as we integrate GenAI into clinical practice, we must carefully consider its impact on the doctor-patient relationship and the delicate art of understanding illness. While the technology offers exciting possibilities for improving diagnosis and information accessibility, it also raises questions about the nature of medicine itself. If we limit our understanding of GenAI to its role as an information provider, we risk overlooking its potential to reshape – for better or worse – the human interactions at the heart of medicine, particularly the processes of communication and shared meaning making that are fundamental to a patient's journey.

How does GenAI relate to questions of meaning?

The rise of GenAI in healthcare raises questions about the nature of medicine itself, challenging long-held assumptions about the doctor-patient relationship and the subtle process of understanding illness. Dr. Iona Heath, a respected GP and advocate for a more humanistic approach to medicine, offers a valuable framework for navigating these complexities. She argues that the GP serves a crucial role as a 'gatekeeper' between illness (Heath, 2018) – the patient's subjective experience of suffering – and disease – a medicalised diagnosis that often leads to a specific treatment pathway. The GP, in this view, is not simply a dispenser of diagnoses or prescriptions, but a skilled listener and interpreter, helping patients navigate the often ambiguous terrain of health and illness, recognising the inherent sense of self-vulnerability (Delacroix, 2022) that patients often experience when seeking help. This gatekeeper role, however, faces a new challenge in the age of GenAI. While patients have always sought information about their health, the rise of sophisticated AI-powered tools could significantly renegotiate the power dynamics within the consulting room. This shift in authority could have profound implications for the doctor-patient relationship, eroding trust and diminishing the importance of narrative understanding.

The intrusion of technology into the once-sacred space of the consulting room, where focused attention and empathetic listening were paramount, is not a new phenomenon. As earlier generations of digital tools became increasingly integrated into clinical practice, the doctor-patient relationship was often disrupted, the machine demanding data input and generating standardised outputs at the expense of genuine human connection. GenAI, with its ability to process information at an unprecedented scale, risks dominating the clinical encounter, potentially obscuring the path towards deeper understanding in favour of quick answers and standardised approaches.

The potential for the algorithm's voice to overshadow the patient's narrative points to a broader and more concerning trend: the distillation of human experience into algorithmic pronouncements. GenAI, in its pursuit of efficiency and objectivity, risks reducing the patient's story, that tangled skein of memory, emotion and lived experience, to a neat set of data points (Figure 8.2).

This streamlining of suffering, where complexity is flattened into diagnostic codes and treatment algorithms, risks obscuring the very human dimensions of illness that Illich so eloquently championed: the subjective experience of pain, the social and cultural contexts that shape our understanding of health, and the individual's capacity for resilience and self-healing.

Consider, for example, a patient presenting with fatigue, anxiety and difficulty sleeping. A GenAI-powered diagnostic tool might efficiently point towards generalised anxiety disorder. But what if their weariness stems from something that defies easy categorisation – the burden of a recent loss, the ache of a broken relationship, or the quiet despair of a life that feels out of sync with their deepest values? What if their sleeplessness is less a symptom of a diagnosable condition, and more a sign of a soul struggling to find its bearings in the darkness?

When an AI excels in language, as GenAI demonstrably does, it offers the potential to enhance communication and understanding in healthcare. Imagine a GenAI system that can help patients articulate their experiences more effectively, ensuring their voices are heard and their needs are met. However, this potential must be carefully balanced against the risk of GenAI silencing the very narratives it aims to support. The 'textures of the patient's experience' – the raw, unquantifiable elements that make their suffering so uniquely their own – risk being overlooked when the algorithm takes centre stage. The danger is that the patient's story,

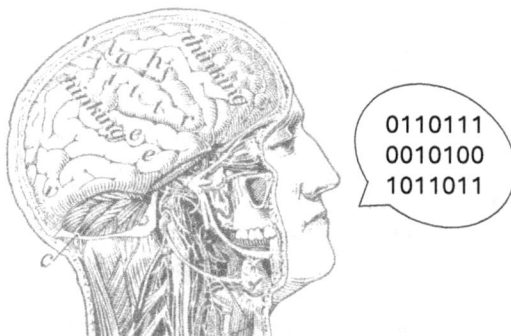

Figure 8.2 Distillation of Human Experience to Data Points (Clark, 2009).

instead of being the starting point for a shared exploration of meaning and healing, becomes merely a source of data to be fed into the machine. The doctor, guided by the algorithm's assessment, might inadvertently miss the deeper story, the unspoken fears and hopes that lie beneath the surface of the patient's words. Furthermore, the very act of relying on GenAI to generate patient narratives and suggest diagnoses could subtly shift the doctor's role, potentially leading to 'diagnostic laziness' and a gradual erosion of clinical judgement and interpretive skills. The art of medicine, honed through years of experience and careful observation, risks being overshadowed by the allure of algorithmic certainty.

The 'medical gaze,' a concept developed by the French philosopher Michel Foucault, highlights a subtle yet profound way in which GenAI might impact our experience of health and illness. Foucault argued that medicine's power lies not just in its ability to cure disease, but also in its ability to define what constitutes normality and deviance. This power to define, he suggested, shapes not only how we are seen by others, but also how we see ourselves. GenAI, with its capacity for constant monitoring and analysis, could amplify this 'gaze,' influencing our self-perception and our relationship with our bodies in ways we might not even be aware of. Imagine wearable sensors tracking our every heartbeat, sleep cycle, and mood fluctuation, feeding data into algorithms that generate personalised assessments and recommendations. This constant scrutiny could lead to a hyper-medicalised view of ourselves, where every variation from the statistical norm is viewed as a potential problem requiring intervention.

The amplification of the 'medical gaze' through GenAI highlights a paradox: the pursuit of greater control over our health might inadvertently diminish our capacity for embracing the uncertainties and complexities of human experience. The 'art of not knowing' involves a willingness to tolerate ambiguity, to resist the allure of easy answers, and to recognise that healing often unfolds in unexpected ways. GenAI, with its reliance on data and algorithms, could inadvertently push us towards a more mechanistic and less holistic understanding of health, potentially obscuring the wisdom that can be found in the spaces between certainty and doubt.

How can patients and doctors use GenAI to discuss the meaning of illness, values and choices of interpretation and action?

The previous sections have highlighted the potential risks of GenAI in healthcare, particularly its potential to streamline suffering, extend the medical gaze, and prioritise algorithmic certainty over the nuanced complexities of the doctor-patient relationship. However, this technology also offers opportunities for enhancing communication, deepening understanding and fostering a more collaborative and patient-centred approach to care.

One way to envision GenAI's potential is as a bridge between the technical world of medicine and the lived experience of illness. Consider the moment when a patient, newly diagnosed with a complex condition, struggles to grasp the technical language used to explain their illness. The doctor, sensing the patient's apprehension, could turn to GenAI to generate a personalised summary of the diagnosis,

transforming medical jargon into clear, concise language that the patient can readily understand. Unlike traditional online resources, which can often leave patients
feeling overwhelmed and uncertain (Abdelghani et al., 2024), GenAI offers the
potential for a more personalised and tailored dialogue that empowers patients to
make informed decisions. This bridging act not only provides access to information but also creates a space for deeper dialogue, where patients can ask informed
questions, engage more fully in discussions about treatment options, and ultimately
feel more in control of their health journey.

In the realm of shared decision-making, GenAI can act as a bridge, not just
between the quantifiable aspects of risk and the subjective nuances of the patient's
experience, but also between the complexities of medical research and the patient's
own understanding. When facing a difficult choice between treatment options, a
patient needs more than just statistics and probabilities. They need a way to make
sense of the often-intimidating language of clinical trials, to weigh potential outcomes and side effects against their own values and preferences. GenAI can help
facilitate this process, translating technical jargon into clear, concise language,
acknowledging the limitations of 'guideline-based medicine,' and emphasising the
importance of individual patient values. It can foster a more balanced conversation, one where medical expertise and patient preferences are given equal weight.
However, shared decision-making demands more than just presenting options; it
requires clinicians to remain attuned to the patient's individual hopes, fears and
beliefs, recognising that these subjective factors might not be fully reflected in the
data presented by GenAI.

To illustrate this point, consider two scenarios: a patient advised to undergo a
risky but potentially life-saving surgery and a patient with a chronic pain condition who is hesitant to start a new medication due to concerns about potential side
effects. While GenAI might efficiently calculate the statistical probability of success and survival in the first case or highlight the low probability of side effects
in the second, it might overlook crucial subjective factors: for example, the first
patient's deep-seated fear of hospitals, their spiritual beliefs about life and death,
or their desire to spend their remaining time with loved ones rather than undergo-
ing gruelling treatment. And it might overlook the second patient's previous negative experiences with medications, their mistrust of the pharmaceutical industry, or
their preference for alternative therapies. These are not easily quantifiable factors;
yet, they are essential to understanding the meaning of risk for each individual
patient and ensuring their values are respected in the decision-making process.

This highlights a key challenge of GenAI in the realm of risk: the very act of
quantifying and measuring, while seemingly objective, can obscure the subjective,
nuanced, and often unquantifiable aspects of human experience. The patient's story,
their values, their hopes, and their fears – these are the threads that weave together the
fabric of meaning, and these are the threads that the algorithm might miss.

Could GenAI offer a way to address this very challenge? Could it, perhaps,
serve as a bridge not just between data and experience but also between the clinical
encounter and the patient's life beyond the consulting room? Could an AI companion help patients narrate and reflect on their experiences of health and illness,

capturing their concerns, goals, and values in a way that can be seamlessly integrated into the doctor's understanding. This AI companion might provide a comprehensive report before or after a patient visit, ensuring that all parties involved in the conversation are fully informed and that the patient's voice is central to the decision-making process.

The very structure and flow of the consultation might shift in the presence of GenAI. Instead of a clinical encounter dominated by screens and data entry, we might see the emergence of a space where conversation and examination again take centre stage. Perhaps a whiteboard screen on an empty wall, summoned by voice, would replace the ubiquitous computer monitor, displaying relevant information like those old 'white-light boxes' for X-rays. In a world where technology often amplifies noise and distraction, GenAI offers the possibility of creating space for silence in the clinical encounter. By taking on some of the informational and technical tasks – generating summaries, clarifying complex concepts, providing access to research – the technology could free up both doctor and patient to simply be present with each other, fostering deeper listening, reflection, and connection. This shared silence, far from being empty, could become a 'third space' of meaning making, where the algorithm's insights and the human touch intertwine to foster new understandings of illness and healing.

Within this space of shared silence, the very structure of the clinical encounter might subtly transform, with new patterns of interaction emerging that anthropologist Victor Turner might recognise as rituals – symbolic actions that create a sense of order, meaning, and transition – much like the experience of illness itself (Kapferer, 2019).The structured use of GenAI – the inputting of symptoms, the generation of reports, the sharing of information – could become part of a more intuitive and less formalised flow within the consultation. This shift could foster a sense of shared purpose and understanding, creating a more collaborative and less hierarchical relationship between doctor and patient. However, even as these new patterns offer a sense of order and clarity, we must be mindful that they retain the potential to overshadow the individual needs and experiences of the patient.

GenAI might also offer a new avenue for the doctor's own reflective practice, one that echoes the insights gained in Balint groups (Balint, 1955; Horder, 2001). These groups, where clinicians gather to discuss challenging cases and explore their emotional responses, have been shown to provide valuable support, foster resilience and even reduce burnout among physicians, benefits particularly crucial in today's demanding healthcare environment. By engaging with GenAI, doctors could potentially use the technology as a sounding board (Lewis & Hayhoe, 2024), a partner in the process of meaning making that complements traditional forms of reflection. However, this reliance on technology for such a personal and professionally formative process also raises questions about over-reliance and the potential for bias in AI-generated insights. To mitigate these risks and ensure that GenAI supports rather than hinders reflective practice, continuous feedback and refinement from the wider clinical community will play a crucial role (Delacroix, 2024). Furthermore, while offering new avenues for reflection, GenAI could also exacerbate a busy clinician's isolation if it becomes a substitute for seeking support and connection with colleagues. While GenAI can offer valuable perspectives, it's important to remember that technology cannot fully replicate the depth and complexity of human interaction that is so essential to ethical and compassionate care. This vision of GenAI as a facilitator of dialogue, a bridge for complex concepts, a creator of space for reflection, and a potential catalyst for new rituals aligns with the hope, expressed in the introduction, that technology, when guided by human values, might awaken to its potential as a powerful ally in the quest for a more humane and compassionate healthcare system.

Opportunities and perils

The integration of GenAI into healthcare presents a profound paradox: the pursuit of greater control over our health through data and algorithms might inadvertently diminish our capacity for embracing the uncertainties and complexities of human experience. As we've suggested, the very technologies that promise to liberate us from suffering could also confine us within a narrow, technologically mediated view of well-being, where every deviation from the statistical norm is seen as a problem to be solved.

This tendency towards over-medicalisation is further amplified by the current limitations of AI systems themselves. Their propensity always to generate an output, even when faced with uncertainty or ambiguity, coupled with the potential for them to prioritise user satisfaction and confirmation over objective truth, can create a feedback loop that reinforces existing societal biases, echoing the 'echo chamber' effect often observed in social media. The danger lies in the potential for these systems to create a false sense of certainty, prioritising what's 'most likely to be liked' by users over a nuanced understanding of the complexities and uncertainties inherent in medical knowledge, especially as these systems evolve and their underlying logic becomes less transparent. Furthermore, in a system driven by liability concerns, AI companies might be compelled to design systems that err on the side of caution, potentially leading to an over-medicalisation of everyday experiences. This could manifest in increased referrals to specialists, unnecessary tests and treatments, and a diminished role for the cautious judgement and watchful waiting approach that often characterises skilled primary care.

Despite these concerns, the emergence of LLMs offers a potential pathway towards a more balanced and nuanced approach to AI in healthcare. Unlike previous AI tools, or 'cultural technologies' (Yiu et al., 2023), which often led to a more fragmented and depersonalised approach to care, LLMs offer us a digital interlocutor capable of sustaining a conversation. This conversational ability, resonant with the hermeneutic focus on dialogue and interpretation, could lead to a different view of understanding the patient's narrative and lived experience, moving beyond the limitations of information delivery. Currently, many LLMs are designed primarily to generate outputs that users are likely to find agreeable or confirming. However, the underlying mechanisms that shape these outputs can be recalibrated to foster a heightened awareness of the specific context. Just as earlier generations of digital tools introduced unforeseen challenges into the clinical encounter, GenAI, despite its advancements, requires thoughtful integration and human guidance to avoid repeating past mistakes. For instance, an LLM could be designed to accompany its suggested diagnostic tests for a clinical presentation with a pop-up such as 'My analysis is based on the information entered, but remember that I haven't examined the patient. Consider if there are any unspoken concerns or subtle findings that might need further exploration.' Or, if the LLM is listening in on the consultation, it might flag subtle cues of misunderstanding or unmet needs and encourage the doctor to explore these areas more deeply.

GenAI, with its unprecedented access to knowledge and its ability to generate personalised insights, offers both opportunities and challenges in our pursuit of a more holistic understanding of healing. While it might empower individuals to take a more active role in managing their health and provide access to a wider range of treatment options, it also risks reinforcing a narrow, technocratic view of well-being, one that prioritises measurable outcomes over the subjective realities of human experience. The task before us is to ensure that GenAI serves the broader goals of healthcare, not just its technical aims. We must resist the temptation to reduce healing to a purely technical process, remembering that the human journey through illness is complex, unpredictable and deeply personal.

Criteria for maturity and safety

As GenAI enters the realm of healthcare, a crucial question arises: how can we ensure that this powerful technology enhances, rather than diminishes, the human element of medicine? The authors, reflecting on decades of experience witnessing the evolution of technology in healthcare, caution against uncritical embrace of innovation. Earlier generations of digital tools, while promising efficiency and progress, often brought unforeseen challenges – the intrusion of machines into the once-sacred space of the consulting room, the standardisation of patient narratives and the allure of algorithmic certainty that sometimes overshadowed the messy realities of human suffering.

To navigate the uncharted territory of GenAI, we need to learn from both the successes and the failures of the past. Traditional evaluation criteria, while essential for ensuring accuracy, reliability, and safety, represent only one piece of the puzzle when it comes to assessing GenAI's impact. These tools, with their ability to engage in dialogue and adapt to user feedback, offer a unique opportunity for collaboration and shared learning. We need to move beyond simply evaluating GenAI against a checklist and embrace a more dynamic approach, working hand-in-hand with clinicians, patients and other stakeholders to ensure these tools are continuously refined and improved based on real-world experience. This participatory approach is vital if we want GenAI to truly serve the goals of healthcare, fostering a more humane, equitable and patient-centred system (Delacroix, 2024).

Accuracy and reliability are paramount. Any medical technology must provide trustworthy information, especially in the contexts of diagnosis, treatment recommendations, and patient education. Rigorous testing and validation are essential, ensuring that GenAI systems align with established medical knowledge and best practices. Early diagnostic coding systems, as the author observed, often led to inaccurate or misleading labels being attached to patients, with potentially detrimental consequences for their care. Such errors must be avoided with GenAI, demanding the highest standards of accuracy and reliability. In this light, hallucination is still an ongoing concern with AI models (Farquhar et al., 2024).

Bias mitigation and fairness must be addressed with unwavering vigilance. AI algorithms are often trained on data that reflects existing biases and inequalities in society, potentially leading to GenAI systems that perpetuate or even exacerbate health disparities. These biases must be identified and mitigated, ensuring that GenAI applications are fair and equitable for all patients, regardless of background, ethnicity, or socioeconomic status. This requires careful data curation and algorithm design, as well as ongoing monitoring and evaluation to address any emerging biases.

Transparency and explainability are also crucial. The 'black box' problem, where AI's decision-making processes remain opaque and difficult to understand, undermines trust and accountability in healthcare. Clinicians need to understand how GenAI arrives at its conclusions, and patients deserve clear explanations for the recommendations they receive. Transparency is essential not only for building trust, but also for ensuring that clinicians retain their role as the primary interpreter of the patient's experience, guided by both data and human judgement. While the explainability of decisions might be limited for certain AI models, recent progress has been made by providing an overview of the 'reasoning process' during the generation of answers. Additionally, transparency could be achieved by providing a clear indication of the provenance of training data, which would help assess the potential for biased interpretations.

Privacy and data security are non-negotiable in the age of AI-driven healthcare. GenAI systems rely on vast amounts of patient data, raising legitimate concerns about confidentiality and security. Robust safeguards are essential to prevent unauthorised access, breaches, and misuse. Patients need assurance that their sensitive health information is being protected and their privacy respected. Clear guidelines, strong legal frameworks, and a commitment to ethical data handling practices are vital. Current AI models are also incredibly expensive and costly to run, given the computational costs implied, and therefore information has to 'leave' the consulting room, with the potential for abuse and misuse. While it is possible to envisage that more computing power will make these AIs possible to be run locally, it is likewise probable that model complexity will continue to increase, so they will still require some form of remote server facilities that must comply with the strictest levels of data protection.

Finally, and perhaps most importantly, *human oversight and control* must be paramount. While GenAI can offer powerful tools for analysis, interpretation, and communication, it should never replace the clinician's judgement, empathy, or the human connection at the heart of medicine. The allure of technological solutionism must be resisted, ensuring that GenAI systems augment, not replace, human capabilities. Ongoing education and training for clinicians, clear ethical guidelines and a commitment to a patient-centred approach, where technology serves the goals of medicine, not dictates them, are essential.

It is still unknown how the use of AI assistance will impact healthcare professionals cognitively. At the same time as we may delegate some of the most arduous and clerical tasks to AIs, the potential of AI to provide reasoning support entails the risk of making doctors pay 'less attention to detail.'

These criteria, shaped by the authors' experience and the broader ethical and hermeneutic concerns we've explored, offer a framework for navigating the complex landscape of GenAI in healthcare. The integration of this powerful technology into medicine requires a cautious and thoughtful approach, one that prioritises accuracy, transparency, fairness, privacy and human oversight. Only then can we hope to harness the potential of GenAI to enhance our capacity for care, understanding, and connection, ensuring that the future of medicine remains deeply rooted in the human heart.

Agenda for education, dissemination, implementation and research

The integration of GenAI into healthcare is not a distant future scenario; it's a reality unfolding before us. The choices we make today will determine whether this technology enhances or diminishes our capacity for care, understanding, and connection. We must move beyond simplistic pronouncements of either utopian promise or dystopian doom and engage in a thoughtful and proactive dialogue about how to shape the future of AI in medicine. We must not neglect unintended consequences and second order effects: as with any new technology, they will likely appear.

This calls for a multi-faceted agenda, one that addresses the needs and perspectives of clinicians, patients, ethicists, technology developers, policymakers and the broader public. It's an agenda that embraces both the potential benefits and the inherent risks of GenAI, acknowledging the need for careful guidance, continuous evaluation and a commitment to human-centred values.

The introduction of GenAI into healthcare demands a shift in medical education. We need to cultivate a new generation of clinicians who are not just experts in data analysis, but also skilled listeners, astute interpreters of narratives, and sensitive navigators of the complex emotional and existential dimensions of illness. This requires a curriculum that goes beyond the traditional biomedical model, incorporating the humanities – literature, philosophy, history and the arts – to foster a 'hermeneutic sensibility' among doctors. By immersing future clinicians in the rich tapestry of human experience, we can equip them to engage with patients not just as data points, but as whole persons, recognising the unique stories, values, and aspirations that shape their understanding of health and illness.

The future of AI in healthcare should not be dictated solely by Big Tech. We need to create more space for open-source platforms, community-based initiatives and patient-led research projects, empowering individuals and communities to participate more actively in shaping the development and implementation of GenAI. This democratisation of AI development would ensure that these technologies reflect diverse values and priorities, addressing the needs of marginalised populations and challenging the dominance of profit-driven motives. Imagine a world where patients are not just passive recipients of AI-driven healthcare, but active collaborators in its design, ensuring that it aligns with their needs, values and aspirations. Likewise, we need to ensure that as our health systems are updated, clear and useful regulation is introduced, both to harness the potential of AI, and prevent its misuse.

Furthermore, we need to rethink how we measure the success of GenAI in healthcare. Instead of solely focusing on traditional metrics like efficiency and cost-effectiveness, we should develop a broader set of measures that capture the human impact of this technology (Coiera & Fraile-Navarro, 2024). How does GenAI affect patient satisfaction, the quality of communication, and the level of trust in the doctor-patient relationship? Does it enhance or diminish the patient's sense of agency and empowerment? Does it contribute to a greater sense of meaning and purpose in the face of illness? By prioritising these humanistic and existential outcomes, we can ensure that GenAI serves the broader goals of healthcare, not just its technical aims.

Finally, we must foster a culture of *critical AI literacy* among both clinicians and the public. This involves teaching people how to identify and critically evaluate AI-generated information, understand the limitations of algorithms and engage in informed discussions about the ethical and societal implications of this technology. We need to empower individuals to become discerning users of AI, recognising both its potential benefits and its inherent risks. This critical literacy will be crucial for ensuring that GenAI is used responsibly and ethically, in a way that enhances rather than diminishes our shared humanity.

This agenda, while ambitious, is essential for navigating the complex landscape of AI in healthcare. The integration of GenAI into medicine requires a profound shift in perspective, one that recognises the interdependence of technology and humanity. The task before us is to ensure that GenAI serves the broader goals of healthcare, not just its technical aims. We must resist the temptation to reduce healing to a purely technical process, remembering that the human journey through illness is complex, unpredictable and deeply personal. The future of medicine depends not on our ability to conquer disease through algorithms, but on our capacity for empathy, compassion and the kind of wisdom that emerges from embracing the uncertainties of life.

References

Abdelghani, R., Wang, Y.-H., Yuan, X., Wang, T., Lucas, P., Sauzéon, H., & Oudeyer, P.-Y. (2024). GPT-3-driven pedagogical agents to train children's curious question-asking skills. *International Journal of Artificial Intelligence in Education, 34*(2), 483–518. https://doi.org/10.1007/s40593-023-00340-7

Adler-Milstein, J., Zhao, W., Willard-Grace, R., Knox, M., & Grumbach, K. (2020). Electronic health records and burnout: Time spent on the electronic health record after hours and message volume associated with exhaustion but not with cynicism among primary care clinicians. *Journal of the American Medical Informatics Association, 27*(4), 531–538.

Balint, M. (1955). The doctor, his patient, and the illness. *The Lancet, 265*(6866), 683–688.

Bender, E. M., Gebru, T., McMillan-Major, A., & Shmitchell, S. (2021). On the dangers of stochastic parrots: Can language models be too big? In *Proceedings of the 2021 ACM conference on fairness, accountability, and transparency*.

Clark, S. (2009). *Our brain* (Image of page from book published in 1909; edited with digital speech bubble added by Robert Clarke in 2025). Wikimedia Commons. https://commons. wikimedia.org/wiki/File:Pg_226_Our_Brain.jpg

Coiera, E., & Fraile-Navarro, D. (2024). *AI as an ecosystem—Ensuring Generative AI is safe and effective* (Vol. 1, p. AIp2400611). Massachusetts Medical Society.

Delacroix, S. (2022). Professional responsibility: Conceptual rescue and plea for reform. *Oxford Journal of Legal Studies, 42*(1), 1–26.

Delacroix, S. (2024). *Lost in conversation? Hermeneutics, uncertainty and large language models.* Social Science Research Network. https://doi.org/10.2139/ssrn.4751774

Farquhar, S., Kossen, J., Kuhn, L., & Gal, Y. (2024). Detecting hallucinations in large language models using semantic entropy. *Nature, 630*(8017), 625–630.

Hacklai, Y. (2019). *Plato and Aristotle: Dialectics by Luca della Robbia* (Photo). Wikimedia Commons. https://w.wiki/EZUn

Heath, I. (2018). *Matters of life and death: Key writings.* Routledge.

Horder, J. (2001). The first Balint group. *The British Journal of General Practice, 51*(473), 1038.

Illich, I. (1975). *Medical Nemesis: The expropriation of health.* Pantheon Books.

Kapferer, B. (2019). Victor turner and the ritual process. *Anthropology Today, 35*(3), 1–2. https://doi.org/https://doi.org/10.1111/1467-8322.12502

Lewis, M., & Hayhoe, B. (2024). The digital Balint: Using AI in reflective practice. *Education for Primary Care*, 1–5. https://doi.org/10.1080/14739879.2024.2372606

Microsoft Prensa. (2023). *Madrid health service, a pioneer in applying generative artificial intelligence to improve diagnosis for patients with rare diseases.* Retrieved 24/10/2024 from https://news.microsoft.com/es-es/2023/09/15/madrid-health-service-a-pioneer-in-applying-generative-artificial-intelligence-to-improve-diagnosis-for-patients-with-rare-diseases/

Pal, A., & Sankarasubbu, M. (2024). Gemini goes to med school: Exploring the capabilities of multimodal large language models on medical challenge problems & hallucinations. *arXiv preprint arXiv:2402.07023.*

Saab, K., Tu, T., Weng, W.-H., Tanno, R., Stutz, D., Wulczyn, E., Zhang, F., Strother, T., Park, C., & Vedadi, E. (2024). Capabilities of gemini models in medicine. *arXiv preprint arXiv:2404.18416.*

Yiu, E., Kosoy, E., & Gopnik, A. (2023). Imitation versus Innovation: What children can do that large language and language-and-vision models cannot (yet)? *arXiv preprint arXiv:2305.07666.*

9   Hermeneutic approaches to leadership

Jo-Anne Johnson and Sanjiv Ahluwalia

Leadership philosophy and its practice are heavily contested in academic literature. It is clear however that leadership style has significant impacts on patient care, staff experience and ultimately the effectiveness of our health and care system. In this chapter, we explore the current context of leadership in the NHS, and using case studies, how a hermeneutic approach to leadership practice can influence better patient and staff experience.

Organisational change in the NHS

With the advent of the Thatcher government in the 1980s, the NHS has been through profound changes in the way it is managed. The rise of managerialism ushered in the 1980s (Griffiths, 1983), the introduction of commissioning and development of the internal market (Department of Health, 1990) and the target-driven culture in the 2000s were followed by the Lansley reforms (Department of Health, 2012) that sought to consolidate the shift towards a performative healthcare system.

Much has been made of the lack of capital funds for the healthcare system, failures in workforce planning, and the shocks of Brexit and COVID on performance and patient outcomes (Darzi, 2024). But the obsession of healthcare leadership and management with structural reform fails to recognise or acknowledge the consequences on the way components of the healthcare system (and those working within it) interact with each other. At various stages, GPs have been pitted against hospital consultants, regulators against service providers, managers against clinicians and patients against health practitioners through a failure of leadership. The wasted opportunities and additional activity emerging from such an adversarial system of checks and balances have meant that collaboration, engagement, relationships and localism have suffered. Clinical leaders have struggled to counter the imbalance created in healthcare systems by near-continuous structural reform.

The fallacy of solutions

A constant refrain is that the reform of healthcare through effective clinical leadership is required to 'permanently fix' the quality and other concerns that emerge in complex systems. For example, despite numerous attempts to resolve the issues

DOI: 10.4324/9781003517665-9

associated with children's social care over the last 30 years, we continue to hear about high-profile failures of health and care systems.

As Valerie Iles (2011) suggests, the best we can hope for when dealing with complex and messy situations is that we will muddle through from one situation to another, and in doing so, we 'might' make the situation a little better, but also generate a range of unforeseen and unforeseeable consequences. In that sense, the idea of leadership as an all-important fixer of system problems is a fallacy. It is more likely that clinical leaders are best placed to develop a deeper understanding of the issues; engage widely, often, and at multiple layers; and adopt a more considered and sceptical disposition, when it comes to demands for 'system-wide' and 'radical' change.

Democratic deficit in health and care leadership

Clinical leaders are often held up as representing a body of workers across health and care and it is assumed that they speak for and on behalf of the workforce. Such a view may result in a neat rationalisation for management structures and it may also make politicians and others feel better that the 'workforce' has been involved in decision-making. However, we suggest that nothing could be further from the truth. The recent Darzi report (2024) is a stark reminder of the significant gap between politicians and the service itself: it lays bare the degree to which the NHS has been allowed to drift from where it needs to be. One can ask where were clinical leaders during the time the NHS was allowed to deteriorate?

It is well-recognised that healthcare systems (and access) play a significant role in patient and population outcomes. Even more significant is the role of other determinants such as housing, education, employment and the environment (Kindig & Stoddart, 2003). Multiple attempts to engage local government in healthcare policy and delivery have taken place over the past few years, but with little success. Indeed, the transfer of the public health budget to local government was meant to link the two – however, capacity and capability have shrunk through cuts to non-NHS departmental finances (Patel et al., 2024).

These factors have eroded the ability of local communities and systems of health and care to make effective decisions based on the needs of their populations. This democratic deficit in the management of health and care resources cannot be made up by using clinical leaders and patient representatives as proxies for profound and significant changes to health and care systems. It cannot replace deep and ongoing engagement with local people, through the hard graft of meaningful dialogue as well as democratic and other processes that form the basis of our local and national governance.

Seeing healthcare as a complex system

Healthcare has been viewed as a machine with fixed, interconnected parts operating through predictable cause-and-effect relationships. Instead, it is better understood as a complex system, where the conventional rules of causality hold limited sway

(Sweeney & Griffiths, 2002). Mandating changes to address perceived 'deficits' in such a system can often result in unintended consequences, potentially causing more harm than good.

In complex systems, diverse components – such as GP surgeries, hospitals, pharmacies and community services – interact dynamically and continuously. These interactions are not merely transactional; they are the breeding ground for innovation and the evolution of effective healthcare practices. However, interactions are influenced by a variety of internal and external factors, such as policy changes, financial incentives and societal expectations. Crucially, the impact of these influences is neither straightforward nor easily discernible. Cause-and-effect relationships in complex systems are often subtle, nonlinear and context-dependent, making outcomes challenging to predict.

As a result, the behaviour of complex systems defies simple forecasts. Changes within the system can produce ripple effects – some beneficial, others detrimental – that emerge unpredictably over time. Recognising healthcare as a complex system requires us to approach reform with humility, appreciating that small, well-intentioned interventions might yield unexpected consequences.

A local healthcare system undertook a significant planning process to redesign paediatric processes. The pressure had built up to do so to meet fiscal gaps, and the perception that there were 'too many' paediatric units. The proposal put forward was to rationalise the number of acute paediatric sites and maternity units.

The proposal was consulted on and led by senior clinicians locally. Despite ferocious opposition from local people, patient groups and frontline clinicians, the proposals were accepted and implemented over several years.

Some years later, quality of care issues emerged in several of the reshaped paediatric and maternity units. Pressure of demand, staff attrition, cultural issues and patient care concerns were increasingly reported. The regional team were concerned enough to intervene and undertook a deep dive analysis of the situation.

Emerging from this analysis were factors such as under-estimating the size of the demand for maternity and paediatric services, difficulties acknowledging the needs of groups difficult to reach (such as refugees and the homeless) and the long-term impact of unknowable events such as Brexit on staff retention.

With these insights, a clinically led team engaged deeply with frontline staff, patient groups, and other groups, to draw up further proposals. At their heart was a strong emphasis on quality of care, patient, and staff experience, and included parts of the healthcare system such as primary, community and mental health as well as the local council, thus mobilising previously unused assets and making the service design more joined up.

New proposals were put forward with broad consensus from across the healthcare system and implemented at pace to resolve the quality of care and staffing issues that had arisen.

Analysis of the case study

In this case study, initial changes to children and maternity services were implemented that made the situation worse rather than better. Factors such as a focus on structural change, the poor quality of patient and staff engagement and the application of linear solutions generated further challenges, warranting high-level intervention from regional and national teams. In response, the leadership team developed an approach recognisable as hermeneutic: one that shifted the lens towards seeing paediatric and maternity services as a part of a larger, more complex system; that attempted deeper engagement with patients, staff and communities; and that focused on quality of care and patient experience as the primary drivers for change, genuinely capturing insights from clinicians working within the system, with a focus on helping others to see the benefits and need for significant change to services through consensus.

Nature of leadership in complex systems

Performative approaches to leadership often fail to address the complexities of 'wicked problems' in healthcare (Rittel & Webber, 1973). They tend to overlook existing assets, exclude vulnerable populations, and rely on linear thinking, focusing on predictable cause-and-effect relationships, intolerance of uncertainty, and the assumption that outcomes can always be measured, predicted, and mitigated. In contrast, effective leadership in complex systems requires a radically different mindset: one that tolerates uncertainty, acknowledges the unpredictability of outcomes and prioritises building on strengths rather than focusing solely on deficits.

There is limited empiric literature on leadership tailored to the realities of complex healthcare systems. Leadership in these settings often wields less influence than is commonly assumed, especially given the inherent unpredictability and interconnectedness of the system (Iles & Ahluwalia, 2015). While clinical leaders must still respond to demands for explanations of poor performance, financial constraints or individual practitioner concerns, their greater challenge lies in improving interactions between system components rather than engaging in continuous structural overhauls. This systems-focused approach, one that values relationships and collaboration, could significantly transform healthcare delivery, particularly within the NHS.

A critical insight into leadership in complex systems is that outcomes are inherently difficult to predict, and cause-and-effect attributions are often misleading. Leaders must navigate high levels of uncertainty while managing unpredictable service designs and changes. These uncertainties often lead to anxiety, not only for the leaders themselves but also for those who look to them for clarity and direction. Chief Medical Officers (CMOs) and Chief Nursing Officers (CNOs) face immense challenges in maintaining engagement with their workforces while under constant pressure to deliver demanding goals. High turnover in senior roles underscores the toll this pressure takes.

This is where hermeneutic leadership becomes crucial. Leaders in complex systems need to help their teams make sense of the uncertainty and challenges they face. Sense-making leadership, focusing on understanding and interpreting the 'messiness' of complex systems, can help stabilise situations and, in some cases, improve them. Importantly, leaders must recognise when this approach is appropriate and when it is not, requiring a holistic view of the system and the relationships within it.

Creating a culture that values systemic thinking over reactive problem-solving could overcome some of the time constraints typically associated with such an approach. Leaders who help others make sense of their context not only mitigate feelings of hopelessness and burnout but also enhance empathy, productivity and, ultimately, outcomes. At a broader level, such leaders act as conveners, bringing diverse perspectives together to better understand the factors driving change and the potential ripple effects of any intervention. By embracing a hermeneutic approach, clinical leaders expand their toolkit beyond traditional leadership models, enabling them to respond more effectively to the challenges of complexity. This adaptability increases the likelihood of fostering sustainable, meaningful change in healthcare systems.

Knowing when to adopt a hermeneutic approach in leadership

Snowden and Boone (2007) provide a useful framework for understanding different situations and the corresponding leadership styles they demand, which aligns closely with the principles of the hermeneutic window explored in this book. According to Snowdon, leadership responses vary based on the nature of the situation:

- Unforeseen circumstances, such as the London bombings in 2005, require leaders to take decisive action. Novel practices often emerge in these scenarios as individuals, such as A&E consultants responding to an unprecedented crisis, adapt and innovate on the spot.
- Complex situations call for a hermeneutic approach. Here, leadership focuses on fostering dialogue, maintaining ongoing engagement, and facilitating sense-making to navigate uncertainty and interconnected challenges effectively.
- Complicated tasks, like designing and building an airplane, demand a structured leadership style. In these cases, success depends on careful planning, adherence to timelines, meticulous attention to detail and precise management of activities.

In healthcare, clinicians almost always operate within emergent or complex scenarios. The day-to-day reality involves grappling with varying degrees of uncertainty, ambiguity, and 'mess.' Leaders in this context have a critical role in helping clinicians make sense of this complexity. Rather than offering rigid solutions, they guide teams in interpreting and understanding their environments, enabling them to respond thoughtfully and effectively to ever-changing challenges.

Operationalising a hermeneutic approach to leadership in teams

Just as the hermeneutic window is a valuable tool in clinical decision-making, it can be applied to clinical leadership, particularly in times of uncertainty, competing external pressures and complexity. In traditional leadership models, often used in clinical practice, the emphasis tends to be on the destination or the overarching

Leader as role model
Leader's use of self
Emotional engagement and connection .
Authenticity and curiosity

Leadership to help navigate uncertainty and complexity
How does a leader influence the culture of the team?
Leadership that notices and mitigates against injustice
How do we influence and interact with external agencie

Hermeneutic leadership

Relational ethical framework
Establishing team values
Exploring purpose and meaning of our work
Exploring and conceptualising professionalism

Reflection on role:
What is my role as a leader here?
What assumptions am I making about the team?
How do my own experiences affect my leadership style?

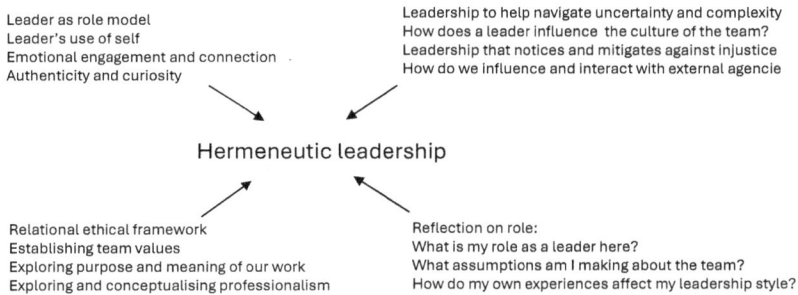

Figure 9.1 Hermeneutic Leadership (Clarke & Shah, 2024).

goal, with a clear focus on the steps needed to reach it. Team members are assigned distinct roles to help navigate the journey, analogous to Snowden and Boone's 'complicated tasks' model. The 'gaze' of the hermeneutic leader shifts from the 'self' to 'the individual' within a team (Figure 9.1).

Using hermeneutics in leadership involves truly seeing, hearing and understanding each team member as an individual. Much like patients presenting with clinical issues in the decision-making model, each team member brings a unique set of experiences, challenges, and perspectives to the table. These personal histories shape their judgements, values, beliefs, problem-solving strategies and interpersonal dynamics within the team. When a leader takes the time to explore a team member's experiences, values and beliefs, the team member themself gains valuable insights into their own strengths, weaknesses and approaches. This reflective process encourages self-awareness and growth. It is only through genuinely understanding each individual team member that a leader can offer the support needed for them to thrive. This approach contrasts with more traditional, authoritarian task-orientated models of leadership often found in clinical settings, where directives are given without regard for individual perspectives.

Hermeneutic leaders must consider their own experiences, values, and beliefs, as these elements shape their leadership style and influence their interactions with team members. External pressures, such as time constraints, can also affect a leader's approach. Being mindful of these influences is essential for collaboratively navigating challenges and finding a path forward.

By empowering team members to take control of their own journeys and fostering self-understanding, leaders help individuals not only achieve their personal goals but also contribute to the team's collective success. This process equips team members with the skills and self-awareness to tackle future challenges independently, ultimately cultivating the next generation of hermeneutic leaders.

Effective team leadership requires understanding how individuals interact and collaborate. However, without a deep appreciation of each team member's unique journey, it can be challenging to gain insight into how individuals function within the team – in terms of both performance and interpersonal dynamics – or to effectively address any team dysfunctions. By adopting a hermeneutic approach, leaders not only gain this understanding but also empower team members to better recognise their own strengths, weaknesses and working styles, as well as that of their colleagues. This awareness fosters improved collaboration and reduces conflict. Through this approach, leaders can guide the team and its members in overcoming challenges – whether solving complex cases, adapting to external factors such as policy changes or resolving internal conflicts. Consider the following case study.

Non-hermeneutic approach

On a busy day in the department, the clinical lead learns that a team member is struggling to meet expectations. Feeling anger and frustration, the lead pulls the individual aside after the ward round to address the issue. They inform the team member that colleagues have raised concerns about their performance, set clear expectations for improvement and caution that failure to meet these standards may lead to formal involvement from Human Resources and their regulatory body.

The team member agrees to the terms and initially meets expectations but soon begins to fall behind again. As the rest of the team faces increased workloads and mounting pressure to meet targets following a recent 'inadequate' departmental rating from the Quality Care Commission, frustration grows among colleagues. Tension escalates within the team, ultimately leading the individual to take an extended period of sick leave.

Hermeneutic approach

On a busy day in the department, the clinical lead is informed that a team member is underperforming. Initially, the clinical lead feels anger and frustration but quickly recognises that this response is unhelpful for both the team and the individual involved. Taking a moment to reflect, they acknowledge that under normal circumstances, one team member struggling would not provoke such a strong reaction.

The lead realises that the team is operating under immense pressure due to new targets introduced after a recent 'inadequate' rating from the Care Quality Commission. These external pressures are likely influencing her own judgement and initial response, as well as the reactions within the team. She schedules a one-to-one meeting with the underperforming team member in a quiet space away from the ward. During the meeting, she takes the time to explore the team member's perspective and any insights they might have regarding their work. The individual admits to struggling to keep up with their work duties and the clinical lead asks for further clarification about the underlying reasons.

The team member tells her that a family member is currently unwell, leaving them feeling overwhelmed and exhausted, which is affecting their work performance. The clinical lead recalls that during prior one-to-one meetings, the team member disclosed significant caregiving responsibilities, which have occasionally made it challenging to balance work and personal life. The lead also remembers that a previous period of leave had been helpful in reducing these pressures and supporting the team member's well-being.

With this context in mind, the clinical lead discusses the situation with the team member, reflecting on their past experiences together. They mutually agree that another period of leave would be beneficial. The lead then holds a meeting with the rest of the team to explain that the individual will be absent for a time, while maintaining confidentiality about personal details. She creates space for the team to share their thoughts and feelings. Concerns about the ongoing quality assurance measures emerge, and the lead helps the team reframe their anger and frustration towards the struggling colleague by acknowledging the broader pressures stemming from these external challenges. The lead collaborates with the team to identify both short-term and long-term adjustments to manage the individual's absence effectively. The team agrees that securing locum cover will be essential to manage workload. In the meantime, they decide that modifying workflows and redistributing roles and responsibilities will provide immediate support. Additionally, the team agrees it would be beneficial to inform the management team about the situation and request a review of their upcoming quality assurance targets to help alleviate external pressures.

After two months, the team member is ready to return to work. The clinical lead arranges a pre-return meeting to evaluate their readiness for reintegration and discusses any necessary adjustments. Additionally, the lead meets with the rest of the team to address any concerns and proactively manage potential challenges before the individual's return. The team has been performing well, meeting their adjusted quality assurance targets.

The team member is gradually reintegrated and their colleagues welcome them back. To ensure ongoing support and monitor progress, the clinical lead conducts regular check-ins with the returning individual. Through one-on-one meetings with other team members, the lead remains attentive to any emerging issues related to the reintegration, including impacts on team dynamics or interpersonal relationships.

Analysis of case study

This case illustrates the reflective nature of hermeneutic leadership and its transformative impact at leadership, team and individual levels. The hermeneutic leader uses reflection to contextualise their initial reaction and recognise their role in addressing the situation.

This self-reflection leads to a shift in thinking and as a result, despite external pressures, the clinical lead prioritises providing the struggling individual with time and space to discuss their challenges. Although the issues raised are at an individual level, the lead recognises the potential for this to affect the whole team's functioning. This individual approach is key to hermeneutic leadership, which reduces the gap between the team leader and their team members. Through the initial one-to-one meeting, the clinical lead explores the individual's level of insight, which is a crucial first step in mutual understanding of the problem and knowing where to begin offering support.

When the team lead draws on a similar past issue and its successful resolution, it fosters a collaborative approach to co-creating a solution, empowering the individual with a sense of control. By working together on the solution, team members not only feel empowered, but also gain valuable tools for addressing similar challenges in the future. By contrast, the alternative non-hermeneutic approach is more direct and solution-focused, emphasising the setting of targets and demands. However, without an understanding of the context of the individual member of staff, inviting and encouraging reflection and the potential for solutions to emerge, it is commonplace for underlying individual issues to remain unaddressed. Negative outcomes for the individual translate into dysfunction both within the team and at personal and functional levels.

Crucially, the lead also creates space for the team to reflect, enabling a shift from initial feelings of anger, frustration, and negative attitudes to the individual concerned, to a shared understanding and collaborative problem-solving. Through this approach, the leader reinforces team values such as compassion and emotional engagement, fostering a more supportive and cohesive work environment.

In this scenario, the team lead's initial reaction mirrored that of the team, but their self-reflection proved valuable in contextualising the team's emotions. The situation could have emerged that one of the team members disagreed with the planned approach, despite the open dialogue and contextualisation. Such disagreements often stem from individual values, which run deeper and are more intricate than initial emotional reactions, but should be explored in the same way, in a listening and understanding approach at the level of the individual. Only through understanding individual values which are shaped throughout a lifetime of an individual's interactions and experiences, will it be possible to mutually agree on a way forward. Furthermore, challenging values within a team can spark new learning and growth, enriching the collective understanding.

Allowing the team to co-create a solution for the planned period of absence of their colleague, ensures that the whole team feels heard and empowered in the process of finding a solution. Providing purpose and meaning for the team is particularly important when navigating times of complexity and uncertainty, for strengthening team relationships, functioning, staff well-being and ultimately improving patient care.

The hermeneutic leadership approach reaches beyond the immediate team. In this instance, the leader uses their insight into the context of the team's concerns and a collaborative, solution-focused approach to effectively mitigate external pressures.

The contrast between the hermeneutic and non-hermeneutic leadership approaches here is clear, with dialogical communication and a focus on sense-making playing a central role. The hermeneutic approach fosters an environment where both the individual and the team feel supported, heard and included in decision-making. Providing time and space for reflection and involving the team in problem-solving is vital for individual well-being and team development and for creating a culture of trust and collaboration.

Concluding comments

In this chapter, we have explored the potential for the use of hermeneutics to inform leadership practice, whether this is at the level of a complex system, within teams, or working with individuals. It is highly likely that leaders work at all these levels and are uniquely placed to see the 'bigger picture.' While a hermeneutic approach is powerful in dealing with complex and often difficult to define situations, it is not the only one that can be taken. It sits alongside such other approaches and each situation requires leaders to carefully consider the most relevant approach to managing change, conflict, and complexity in their specific contexts. Ultimately, leadership itself is challenging, and leaders will benefit from seeking to make sense of their own practice through strategies and techniques that define a hermeneutic approach.

References

Clarke, R., & Shah, R. (2024). *Hermeneutic leadership* (Unpublished illustration).

Darzi, A. (2024). *Independent investigation of the national health service in England.* https://www.gov.uk/government/publications/independent-investigation-of-the-nhs-in-england

Department of Health. (1990). *National health service and community care act* 1990 : *Chapter 19.* Her Majesty's Stationery Office.

Department of Health. (2012). *Health and social care act 2012.* Her Majesty's Stationery Office.

Griffiths, R. (1983). *NHS management inquiry.* DHSS Leaflets Unit.

Iles, V. (2011). *Why reforming the NHS doesn't work: The importance of understanding how good people offer bad care.* Lulu Press.

Iles, V., & Ahluwalia, S. (2015). Clinically led or clinically fronted?: An alternative view of leadership. *British Journal of General Practice, 65*(630), e55–e57.

Kindig, D., & Stoddart, G. (2003). What is population health? *American Journal of Public Health, 93*(3), 380–383.

Patel, N., Gazzillo, A., Vriend, M., Finch, D., & Briggs, A. (2024). *Options for restoring the public health grant.* The Health Foundation. https://www.health.org.uk/reports-and-analysis/briefings/options-for-restoring-the-public-health-grant

Rittel, H. W., & Webber, M. M. (1973). Dilemmas in a general theory of planning. *Policy Sciences, 4*(2), 155–169.

Snowden, D. J., & Boone, M. E. (2007). A leader's framework for decision making. *Harvard Business Review, 85*(11), 68.

Sweeney, K., & Griffiths, F. (2002). *Complexity and healthcare: An introduction.* Radcliffe Publishing.

10 Meaning making in frontline medical education

John Launer and Louise Younie

The importance of enabling patient meaning making and engaging with their wider context has already been argued in this book. Re-narrations, re-interpretations and sense making for patients especially living through poverty, trauma and injustice can be lifechanging. Despite the risk of harm to patients from neglecting these aspects, we still struggle to equip our future and junior colleagues with an education that attends to both diagnosis and meaning making in the consultation.

There are many reasons why enabling medical student engagement in meaning making, their own or their patients, is challenging. These include curriculum focus on technical knowledge, detachment and objectivity, assessment-driven learning, time pressure, lack of role models or structured opportunities and fear of vulnerability and burnout. For clinicians time-pressured, single disease-focused clinical guidelines, expanding knowledge, technology and complexity all serve to reduce space and capacity for engaging in meaning and context in the consultation.

While we recognise the value of technological advances saving many lives in modern medicine, we are concerned about the potential harm and dehumanisation of the individuals working in and engaging with our healthcare systems. In our different ways, the two authors have recognised the challenge and sought to enable meaningful relational human reflection and encounters in both undergraduate and postgraduate spaces. Louise has been introducing creativity and the arts to undergraduate medical education and John has written and taught narrative medicine, in particular an interventive interviewing technique called Conversations Inviting Change, for several decades.

Narrative medicine and conversations inviting change: an introduction

John Launer

I begin my contribution to this chapter by declaring two assumptions. My first assumption is that readers will have some familiarity with medical humanities, the field which attempts to bring understanding and sensitivities from the world of humanities into medicine and hence to humanise practitioners and practice alike. My second assumption is that a large proportion of readers, especially educators in

DOI: 10.4324/9781003517665-10

healthcare, will have an interest in the field known as communication skills. Anyone interested in the search for meaning in medicine is likely to have delivered and almost certainly will have received training in how to listen to patients attentively and to respond with appropriate tact and timing, especially in circumstances such as having to break the news of a serious or incurable illness.

If both my opening assumptions are correct, you may have noticed that there is a puzzling gap or disjunction between these two areas of enterprise. In seminars on reflective writing on medical humanities courses, for example, medical students will commonly be asked to bring personal accounts of patients they have seen on the wards or clinics who have inspired them or caused them distress. Yet I know of no examples where they have also been asked to bring an accompanying video of the clinical conversation that may have taken place, even though video review may be common when learning communication skills. Equally, I am not aware of anyone who has ever invited learners to look at, say, a self-portrait of Frida Kahlo in pain from her multiple orthopaedic problems and then asked someone to act her part in a role play while a volunteer takes her medical history. Although many of us working in what are sometimes dismissively called 'soft skills' may move between teaching medical humanities to one group on a Tuesday morning and communication skills to another group on a Friday afternoon, we still have the peculiar habit of keeping them apart on the curriculum and in our schedules, as if one is too pure to be practical and the other too practical to be pure.

There is one branch of medical humanities that does make an explicit claim for transferability from creative study to clinical communication. It is the branch known as narrative medicine. Emerging at the end of the twentieth century, narrative medicine was a project to bring ideas about narratives or stories, familiar from philosophy and social sciences, into medicine and healthcare. Pioneered in the United Kingdom by two academic general practitioners, Greenhalgh and Hurwitz (1998), and in the United States by the physician and literary scholar Rita Charon (2006), narrative medicine has aimed to counterbalance the dominance of Evidence Based Medicine by pointing out that every patient and every problem requires a response at two levels – that of a solution or outcome, and that of a story or meaning. The case for narrative medicine is simply that without an understanding of how stories are told across all cultures, whether in novels or as presented by patients, our attempts to 'fix' things will very often only be partial. Hence the study of oral and written stories – narratology – is seen as virtually a pre-requisite for humane and ethical practice.

The Chinese scholar of narrative medicine Guo Liping has written the following about medical humanities and narrative medicine:

> The medical humanities are only good at criticizing the 'inhumane' aspects of healthcare and analysing the reasons for such dehumanisation. They are not good at telling and training healthcare professionals HOW to improve their care. Healthcare professionals feel empty-handed and frustrated when facing the unsatisfactory doctor–patient relationship and criticism from the medical humanities yet feel at a loss as to what to do — until they have

narrative medicine… [Narrative medicine is] a willingness on the part of
the clinician to listen to [patients'] stories and respond to their concerns and
needs, and to take actions to alleviate their sufferings the best they can; for
the clinician, it's a willingness to always include the patient's and/or family's
views and life stories in the entire process of healthcare, whether it's in consultation or decision-making, and to take actions to improve the well-being
of the patient (and hence that of the family).

(Guo, 2023)

It is worth noting that before the so-called 'narrative turn' influenced medicine, it
had already penetrated another clinical area – that of mental healthcare where it
was indeed used to make radical alterations in the way some professionals listened
to patients or responded to them. During the second part of the last century, an
increasing number of mental health professionals were moving away from notions
that it was possible to offer definitive interpretations or formulations of mental distress and towards the idea that it was more appropriate and helpful to see the speech
and behaviour of patients as attempts to establish meaning for themselves, The role
of the professional or therapist was therefore often reframed as offering a hermeneutic space in which experiences and feelings could be re-interpreted in a way that
the suffering person found more coherent or effective in conducting their lives and
relationships. This approach came to the fore particularly in therapy with couples
and families, where practitioners often found themselves as witnesses to different
or contradictory accounts of the past or the present from parties in conflict. As a
consequence they realised that their role as professionals was not to judge what was
correct or incorrect, or to claim to offer a superior and more expert account, but to
mediate in a way that allowed shared meaning to emerge, or at least for the parties
to become aware of an irreconcilable distance between their narratives. This shift
led to an emergence of 'postmodern' forms of therapy, including the one created by
Michael White and David Epston that became known as 'narrative therapy' (White &
Epston, 1990). This and similar approaches could be conceptualised as meaning
making or hermeneutic therapy.

Narrative medicine and narrative based practice

When the narrative medicine movement emerged in the late 1990s, I was working
for most of the week as a GP but it so happened that I had also just completed training as a family therapist. I had joined the part time staff at the Tavistock Clinic, a
mental health training institute in north London. As family therapists we already
took the view that our role was not just to help to solve people's problems, but often
to pay close attention to their stories about themselves and each other as well. We
worked with them to try to help them develop stories that offered richer meaning,
more coherence, or more hope. Often, it was our ability to find different meaning in
their problems that helped to improve or resolve the problems themselves.

As a group of colleagues, we felt that there was scope for introducing such ideas
and skills into the practice of medicine, especially in primary care or when dealing

with complex or challenging cases in other specialties. Together with my former tutor, Dr Caroline Lindsey, we decided to set up a course for GPs and primary care nurses (Launer & Lindsey, 1997). One of our aims was also to offer an alternative to so-called Balint groups, which had also been developed at the Tavistock Clinic around 40 years earlier. These were case discussion groups designed to enhance people's sensitivity and awareness of doctor-patient dynamics. In contrast to Balint groups, we wanted to address the whole range of primary care work, including both mental and physical problems, and to teach specific communication skills. We also wanted to address some questions we thought were crucial for primary care. We had a strong belief that ideas about narratives could be helpful in addressing these questions:

- 'How do you practise medicine when the authority of professionals including doctors can no longer be taken for granted?'
- 'How can you share power with patients, without letting go of evidence and science?'
- 'How do you work alongside colleagues who may have other views, other beliefs and other professions?'
- 'How can you practise humanely while following a huge agenda of preventive medicine, disease surveillance, and keeping to guidelines?'
- 'How can you hold on to optimism about the possibility of change when you see so many people who are intractably distressed?'
- 'How can you manage all of this when time and resources are short?'
- 'How can you be a care professional and remain a caring person?'

When ideas about narrative finally began to penetrate medicine as they had done with family therapy, we realised that our project was an attempt to bridge the insights, the moral commitment and the passion of narrative medicine with the needs of health professionals for precise communication skills to apply right across the range of their work. We gave our training the name 'Conversations Inviting Change,' now often abbreviated to CIC. You could conceptualise the relationship between medical humanities, narrative medicine, communication skills and narrative based practice or CIC in terms of the following two diagrams (Figures 10.1 and 10.2).

Figure 10.1 shows CIC as a form of narrative based practice, nesting within the wider field of narrative medicine, which is itself part of the world of medical humanities. Figure 10.2 illustrates how we offer a bridge between narrative medicine and teaching in communication skills (Launer & Wohlmann, 2023). This could be likened to bridging the gap between boxes 3 and 4 in the Four Domain Model (see Figure 10.3).

In the 30 years since we created our courses, our focus has largely been on teaching qualified and established practitioners. Our experience is that such professionals have reached a stage in their careers where they have realised that generic skills and clinical knowledge are not enough to address the complexities that they and their patients face. In some cases, they have hit a wall professionally and are at risk of burnout and are looking for ways of working that will restore meaning for

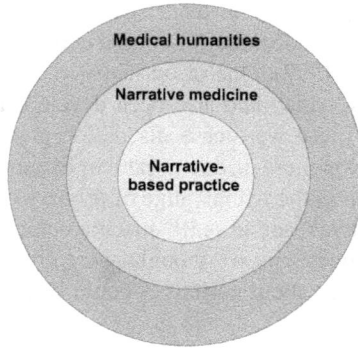

Figure 10.1 Medical Humanities, Narrative Medicine and Narrative Based Practice.

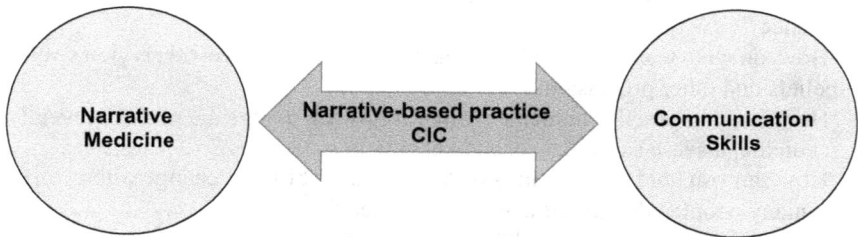

Figure 10.2 Bridging the Gap between Narrative Medicine and Communication Skills.

them, just as we hope to help them fulfil this role for their patients. The underlying principles of our approach remain the same. The first is this:

> Every person's story contains its own momentum for change: good listening and questioning can facilitate this, not by explanation and persuasion but by allowing space for it to develop.

What this means is that you need to approach any patient, student or colleague with faith that any story they tell about themselves has the potential to evolve to another different and better story. You cannot expect to help them get there by 'just listening,' or solely by being a kind and empathic person. You certainly cannot do so by deciding on behalf of the other person exactly where they need to go, by pushing them in that direction, or simply by offering them information and advice. You have to travel as an active companion alongside their story.

Here is the second principle:

> Narrative ideas can be very useful in health care, but they need to be applied in combination with other familiar frameworks including science and evidence. (Boxes 1 and 2 of the Four Domain Model – see Figure 10.3)

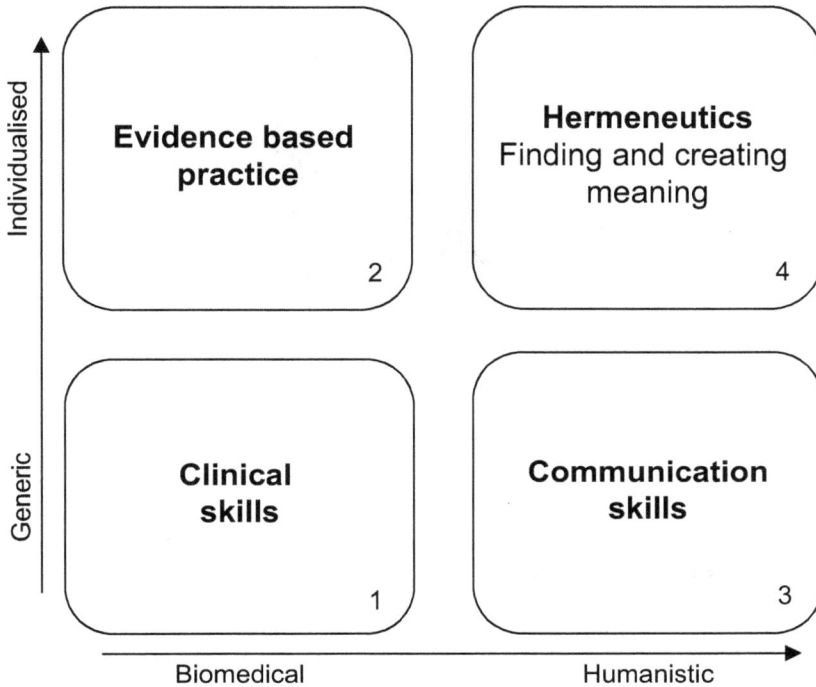

The Four Domain Model, a 2×2 matrix. Vertical axis from "Generic" (bottom) to "Individualised" (top); horizontal axis from "Biomedical" (left) to "Humanistic" (right).

- Top-left box: **Evidence based practice** — 2
- Top-right box: **Hermeneutics** Finding and creating meaning — 4
- Bottom-left box: **Clinical skills** — 1
- Bottom-right box: **Communication skills** — 3

Figure 10.3 The Four Domain Model (Shah et al., 2020).

Medicine and healthcare are not just about stories: they also depend on particular norms regarding science, evidence, safety and professional codes of conduct. As well as having what Rita Charon has called narrative competence – the ability to engage with stories – our patients and our colleagues rightly expect us to be experts and to observe these norms as well. We need technical competence, or what you might call normative competence, as well as narrative competence. You could therefore depict our fundamental tasks as health professionals as in Figure 10.4: it is one that combines narrative practice with norm-based practice or normative practice.

Although the diagram shown here has its origins in the Far East, we use it everywhere, and people understand what it means all over the world. It illustrates that our approach as professionals needs to be balanced between narrative and normative practice, just as the Four Domain Model does. Narrative practice by itself may not help to solve someone's problem, but just following the norms will not do so either, except in a very limited range of cases like surgical emergencies. Almost all the time, patients need to go away with a better story, a better sense of meaning, as well as a treatment or a cure. As the diagram also captures, normative medicine incorporates its own narratives. We realise this, for example, every time the official definition of a condition like ADHD, asthma or hypertension changes and becomes what you might call a new official story. Conversely, patients' narratives

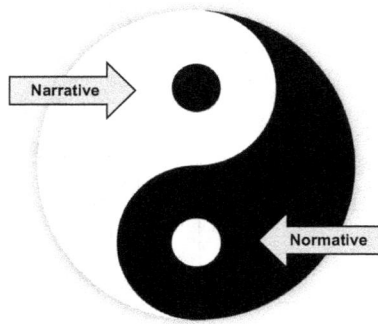

Figure 10.4 Narrative and Normative Practice. Based on Yin and Yang Symbol (Klem, 2007).

may embody medical norms too. For example, a patient might describe symptoms that we instantly recognise to be indications of a serious disease, even if they are unaware of the significance of their words as they speak them.

We teach a range of techniques in 'Conversations Inviting Change' to promote narrative based practice. By far the most important is the skill of questioning. Our belief is that, by enquiring closely into the story brought by patients you gain a much fuller understanding of exactly what the problem is, what meaning it has in the patient's mind, and why exactly it constitutes a problem for them. More important than this, you can also use questions to invite the patient or colleague to examine their own story more critically, and to change their own assumptions about it, or what might be done about it. As I emphasised earlier, this is not a process of persuasion but of shared reflection between practitioner and patient, or practitioner and colleague.

We counsel the people we teach not to learn rigid approaches to questioning, but to develop a style of questioning based on their interest in other people and how each person sees the world around them. But here are the kinds of questions that can be helpful:

Questions we hear in 'Conversations Inviting Change'

What do you see as the main problem or your chief dilemma?
How would you describe it?
What do you think are the main things influencing this situation?
What do I need to know about it?
What explanations do you have for this?
How do you understand it?
What would you like to happen and what do you want yourself?
Who else might have a view about this?
How would they view you/what is going on?
What would they say?
What are the differences here in everyone's beliefs or understanding?

What would happen if you…?
Where do you think things will be in a month or a year…?
Supposing…?
What will happen if nothing changes?

As you may notice, some of these questions are close to the traditional method of taking a medical history. Yet they are also different. The practitioner is focusing not so much on the problem as on the story itself and its meaning to the person telling it. Using this approach, people become very skilled at formulating questions in a way that yields important medical information, while at the same time helping the narrator to reflect on the wider range of influences, for example, family, social or cultural, that have helped to construct the problem to be exactly how it seems to that person.

Narrative based practice in action

When teaching CIC, we nearly always give a demonstration of how we use it in practice. We do this by asking a member of the group to volunteer to bring a narrative concerning an issue or dilemma they are struggling with at work. One of our trained team members will then offer to have a conversation with them about this in front of the whole group of learners. *One of the reasons we nearly always offer such a demonstration is that describing CIC can only give a limited impression of what it involves, particularly with regard to the capacity of practitioners to improvise their questions and elicit quite surprising responses from the narrators.*

On occasion, we also sometimes show a video example of CIC in action. One video I commonly use in this situation shows me holding a consultation with a woman suffering from longstanding severe facial pain. Although the woman is an actor, she has personal experience of the condition, so her performance is highly authentic. The main purpose of the video is to demonstrate how it is often possible to elicit more information – medical as well as biographical – by listening to a story rather than taking a more formal history. In the consultation, I focus from the outset on the patient's family and working context, her love of horses, and the personal impact on these of her persistent pain. In doing so, I find out a great deal in passing about her past medical treatment, her current medication, and what she is seeking by visiting yet another doctor.

Although she begins the consultation by saying 'I want the pain to stop,' she later turns out to be more interested in strategies for living alongside the pain. To the surprise of many who view the recording, it turns out within a few minutes that she isn't requesting more opiates or a further specialist referral, although this seems the case at first. CIC often has this effect, with patients and doctors alike shifting their own perspectives when their stories are given time to breathe. The video itself can be viewed online on the CIC website, where it is framed by an interview with an academic GP colleague and pioneer of hermeneutic approaches to medical practice, Professor Joanne Reeve (Launer, 2024).

Many of the narratives that participants bring to our courses concern dilemmas and tensions in the workplace. These usually relate to the way their teams are functioning or not functioning. They often concern issues of power, interprofessional tensions, differing values, or contrasting attitudes to organisational change. The kinds of ideas and techniques we use are highly relevant to these issues.

I gave an account of one such conversation in the British Journal of General Practice (Bovo & Launer, 2022). I wrote it in collaboration with a young paediatrician from Argentina whom I supervised on a course in CIC. Her career had been impaired by long COVID, but in our conversation she came to the realisation that her medical condition was not the only factor in her distress. It was also the way she had aspired in the past to perfectionism, and in particular to equal a colleague she held up as a role model, rather than pursuing a less ambitious path for her own good and that of her family. These kinds of 'narrative shifts' are common in CIC if you allow someone's story to go where it needs to go.

The most important part of all our trainings takes place in interactive small groups. We break people up into group of four or five where the participants will help each other think about their work – what you could describe as peer supervision. These groups address a problem or dilemma brought by each participant, in turn. One person offers a narrative of something that is bothering them at work: a dilemma with a patient, colleague or team. Another member of the group acts as a peer supervisor, interviewing the narrator about this, using the principles and techniques of CIC. The remaining members of the group act as observers. A trainer monitors the process, introducing pauses in the conversation from time to time and inviting reflections from the interviewer and observers.

There are some similarities here to Balint groups: for example, the group will focus on only one person's narrative at a time, for perhaps 20 or 30 minutes, and these are narratives of real cases and not role play. However, there are significant differences from Balint groups. The main one is that we ask the person acting as an interviewer to try to follow three simple rules in order to learn narrative practice.

- Only ask questions.
- Make sure that each question links directly with something the narrator has already said.
- Withhold any interpretations, suggestions or advice until the end of the conversation.

We have found that this is the only way people can experience directly how hard it is to create a narrative space for someone else, and how liberating it is for everyone when you succeed in doing so. As the course progresses, participants will have a chance to explore how to mix other forms of speech into their conversations. They will learn how to integrate more of their normative approach as health professionals, but for now they must follow these rules.

Conclusion

Through teaching 'Conversations Inviting Change' over many years, we have managed to bring a new view of medical conversations into postgraduate medical training.

In all our teaching, we find it useful to emphasise how a narrative based approach is a horizontal one rather than a vertical one: see Figure 10.5. Rather than digging a deeper and deeper hole every time to try to discover what is at the bottom, we should more often be weaving a tapestry of language with the patient or colleague. They put in a thread, we offer another thread, they add a further thread, with each contribution, and indeed each conversation, making a fabric of meaning. This approach can help clinicians escape the common trap of looking for big problems underneath small ones, or huge problems underneath big ones. More importantly, I think it helps both patients and clinicians to move away from stories of being vulnerable or victims and towards narratives of possibility and agency.

Creative enquiry and meaning making in undergraduate medical education

Louise Younie

The field of medical humanities has been growing in medical education drawing across many areas such as history, philosophy, narrative, literature, music and dance (Anil et al., 2023). In the early days of the arts and humanities movement students predominantly worked with arts and literature produced by others (Milligan & Woodley, 2009). As early adopters we have been inviting students to engage in non-professional creative-reflective approaches for themselves for over the last 20 years (Younie, 2009, 2013, 2014, 2019b). We call this work creative enquiry, which we describe as the process of exploring lived experience through the arts (Younie, 2014). This involves students actually picking up paintbrushes, sketchpads and the camera and creating something which they then write or talk reflectively about and what it means to them.

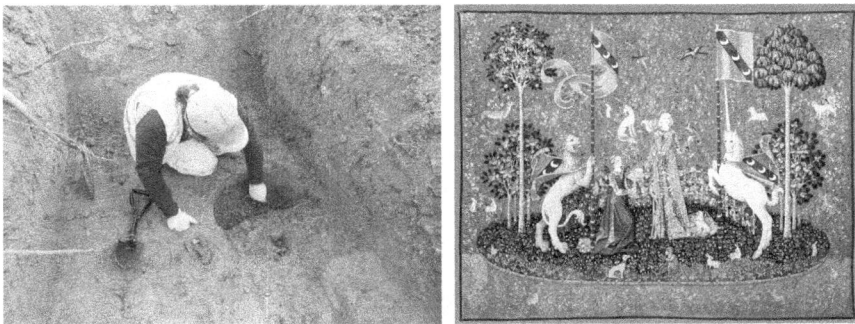

Figure 10.5 Digging a Hole (Hicks, 2023) and Weaving a Tapestry (Descouens, 2021).

We have been drawing on the creative enquiry process to enhance person-centred care and human flourishing in the medical curriculum. Person-centred care and dealing with uncertainty are two of the core tenets of the new Medical Licensing Assessment (MLA) that all medical students will be judged by, alongside knowledge of many different diagnoses. Both person-centred care and uncertainty are challenging to educate for. Bansal et al. (2022), with their realist research into enabling person-centred care in medical education found that teaching objective clinical knowledge within the positivist philosophical framework with additional communication skills, is not enough to enable person-centred care. Person-centred care is not just being nice to the patient, as I thought as a medical student, but demands understanding of the value of enabling agency of the patient and the inherent subjectivity of the clinician. As Bansal et al point out, person-centred care builds on an interpretivist framework. Medical students are in general not interested in the philosophical underpinning; however inviting creative enquiry engagement with lived experience on the wards and in clinics immediately positions the student in a more human, imaginative and curious space.

My journey into creative enquiry as educator started with lived experience as a newly qualified GP where I found that my armoury of diagnoses and treatments was not sufficient. I was unsure how to navigate the complex interpersonal realm so evidently affecting my consultations. How might I do something useful for each patient with their many different hopes, beliefs and concerns and in response to so many clinical presentations with no clear answer, diagnosis or treatment. Initially I felt the pressure of being the big expert with the answers. An experience of a creative writing workshop with Professor Rita Charon about 'a difficult consultation' was transformative. I wrote and reflected on 'the lady in black,' her depression, and how I was rendered helpless in our encounter. In retrospect I realised that I was trying to find as many solutions as possible for *her* in order to make *me* feel better.

When the clinician presents themselves as the only expert or knower in the room, they risk the disempowerment of patient as embodied knower and sense-maker, disrupting the 'creative capacity' of the patient (Carel, 2008). There are similar consequences when an educator, or educational system does the same – the student as knower is denied agency and creative capacity. In a current research study, a student choosing the creative enquiry Student Selected Component (SSC) described their lived experience of medicine this way:

> Medicine… [is] …just memorising, and science based, and I don't feel like there's a lot of … opportunity to think beyond the box… So, I thought it would be a nice break. I think because with medicine you don't really get much time to [engage the] creative side of you. It is more information based and very clinical.

A mirror can be held up between the way we educate our future clinicians and the way in which they treat their future patients. Creative capacity is a concept described by lived experience professor of philosophy Havi Carel (2008), and subsequently through writing and research by professor of primary care research,

Joanne Reeve (2017). Taking these ideas forward into medical education, it might be argued that the concept of 'creative agency' goes beyond person-centred care or student-centred learning in that these terms relate to the doctor or educator endeavouring to do their work in service of the person with less power – the patient or student. However, realising or supporting the creative agency of the other is more akin to lighting a fire with a fire of our own, or releasing something that was always there. In order to enable this kind of creative agency, the clinician or educator must attend to the patient or student and be curious and willing to learn. It means not being obstructed in the relationship by hierarchy or through a colonising approach: by this, I mean imposing rigid, hierarchical structures that prioritise the educator's knowledge, values, and ways of understanding over those of the student (Kinchin, 2023). I am reminded of the following quote by Broyard, cancer patient and editor of the New York Times, where he invites connection between clinician and patient, with the result, not necessarily of the creative capacity of the patient but here perhaps the creative agency of the clinician:

> Not every patient can be saved, but his illness may be eased by the way the doctor responds to him—and in responding to him the doctor may save himself. But first he must become a student again; he has to dissect the cadaver of his professional persona… It may be necessary to give up some of his authority in exchange for his humanity… In learning to talk to his patients, the doctor may talk himself back into loving his work … by letting the sick man into his heart … they can share, as few others can, the wonder, terror, and exaltation of being on the edge of being, between the natural and the supernatural'
>
> (Broyard, 1992, p. 57)

How might we grow clinicians capable, or perhaps willing, at least at times, to engage with this kind of regenerative and nurturing collaborative work alongside traditional history taking, diagnosis and treatment? Creative enquiry may have a role to play.

Over 20 years I have sought to introduce creative-reflective opportunities for medical students to enhance their creative agency within the medical education curriculum. For example, I have developed, run and researched a small group creative arts SSC (Younie, 2013), the bedrock of innovation and learning for me in the field with and alongside students and arts-based facilitators/patient-artists. I have also set up creative-reflective assignments for all year one medical students related to a home visit (Younie, 2009) and on the theme of compassion/generalism for year three medical students (Banu, 2023; Younie, 2022). As a consultant at Anglia Ruskin University I have introduced creative enquiry for the first time into the curriculum, on themes of patient voice, professional identity formation and compassion.

What does a creative enquiry session in medical education look like? The first day of our creative enquiry SSC, for example, involves 12 students and me around a table with creative resources colourfully laid out in the centre of the table. Doodling with the materials is encouraged from the start and students as they arrive may be tasked with finding materials and making some kind of name label, so I can begin to learn names. Small group and large group introductions follow. Students will be introduced to clinical stories, to the materials, to ideas such as patient voice, reflexivity, flow (Czikszentmihalyi, 1990), 'narrative humility' (DasGupta, 2008) and human flourishing (Younie, 2021). They will be given easy creative tasks like drawing breakfast with their eyes closed and sharing, doodling and passing it on, or choosing a postcard. If during the session the students are talking more than the facilitator and talk is directed more towards each other rather than the facilitator, if the students can enter a time of flow and creative silence where they are all exploring through the materials as well as feeling safe enough to begin to share their thoughts around their creation, these feel like the ingredients of a fruitful session. In other SSC sessions, arts for health consultants or arts therapists within differing fields present their way of working, give patient examples, invite students to experience as well as share their creations and emerging questions.

Introducing creative enquiry into medicine has not been easy. I have had to try to find the cracks in the curriculum to scatter and nurture creative seeds (Younie, 2006, 2011, 2014), develop new mark schemes and engage in faculty development and research (Younie, 2006, 2011). The work was sometimes misunderstood at higher levels as commensurate with just going to the theatre in the evening to relax, for example, rather than the collision of creativity and clinical practice to expand practitioner ways of knowing and being alongside patients in their suffering.

Pedagogical affordances of creative enquiry

In the following section, I will explore the ways in which creative enquiry might enable meaning making and relational understanding. My work in the field sits alongside other educators such as Haidet (2007), Shapiro (2009) and Kumagai (2012). Kumagai (2012), for example, introduced student creative-reflective group work around themes emerging from the 'Family Centred Experience' of students encountering patients. He describes three functions of the art. These are art as identity, as critique and interpretation. In the latter conceptualisation, Kumagai explores meaning making and interpretation in three spaces: between students and patient volunteers, across the different students and between students and the art work. He draws on philosophers such as Gadamer (1989) to explore how students encounter patient interpretive horizons and through dialogue and expression seek to make sense of it through their own and their shared artwork.

Through research (Younie, 2006, 2011) and practice, I have boiled down what creative enquiry offers medical education to five key ideas, three of which I present here, including 'meaning making,' 'connection to our interior landscape' and creative enquiry enabling a 'bridge of understanding' with other people. The other two ideas: 'voice' and 'new vistas' are evident throughout the student quotes and images in this section.

Meaning making

Creative enquiry and meaning making are inextricably linked. I have found no better way over the years as a clinical educator, of enabling rich, meaningful conversation around clinical practice and lived experience, than through creative expression. Reflection through the arts enables articulation of our 'meaning schemes' (Polkinghorne, 1988), filled with metaphor, image and emotion. Creative enquiry enables students to capture the language of the human dimension and craft something that may otherwise be difficult to voice. Even doing something as simple as creating a picture that resonates with your lived experience and sharing in groups of three extends our dialogue and sharing. Figure 10.6 shows the idea discussed by one of my students, Sarah Mandourah, on the creative arts SSC and subsequently re-created by artist David Garaway. Sarah wrote about this in the end of course reflection:

> A tree with flowers growing underground on the roots: this was a depiction of how I felt when I first started medical school- isolated, alone and weak. But with time I was able to grow my own roots, and now I cannot be blown over as easily. And these difficult circumstances added colour to my roots, allowing me to see the world through different lenses. Sharing this with other people and saying it out loud made me feel peaceful. I was able to take my pain and make some metaphorical meaning of it. I had carried this around for a long time, the emotional hardships of moving to a new country and being away from my family for the first time and the isolation and loneliness that came with it. And making meaning out of this pain and strife made me feel like I had gained something by going through this difficult experience. I realised if it weren't for these difficult experiences, I wouldn't have my roots and it was not for nothing. I learned that art is not only a form of expression but also meaning. Making connections between different objects and my own feelings and situations helped me not only understand them but also process them and see them from a different point of view.
>
> (Mandourah, 2024)

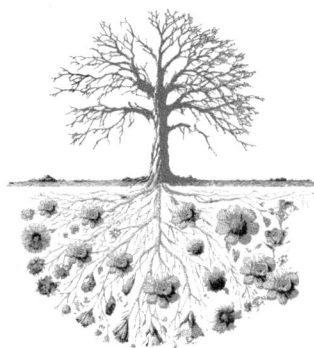

Figure 10.6 A Barren Tree with Flowers Growing on the Roots (© David Garaway, 2025; Used with Permission).

Interior landscape

Students engaging in creative enquiry often describe learning about themselves as one of their core takeaways, being surprised at the extent of their learning. From current research interviews into our creative enquiry SSC as well as reflective writing from longer ago, shared with permission, students say:

> I just learned a lot about myself, and I think that's my main takeaway is that I learned more about myself than I was expecting (Ongoing research into flourishing through creative enquiry, student transcript 13, 2023)
>
> I have enjoyed this SSC because I learnt more about myself in the last two weeks than I have in my twenty-one years. I have been able to open up, when I have always kept my thoughts and feelings to myself.
>
> (Younie, 2019a)

The multi-lingual nature of the arts in creative expression allows a different kind of processing space, rarely found at medical school, but seemingly beneficial:

> The different art forms in the session, including drawing, collage, photography, and poetry all force you to think. To think about the good and the bad, what you can fathom and what is unimaginable. But most importantly it offers a space to process your feelings and life. After 10 weeks of the need to keep going and not fall behind, I was able to take a deep breath in, sit in silence, think about what is happening around me, and try to translate it into a piece of paper. Yes, medicine forces you to think as well, but only in an academic sense, while the art doesn't confine you to any borders.
>
> (M. Kamsad, medical student, personal communication, 2023)

In the following example, medical student Freya Qureshi describes the value of reflection through the non-verbal medium of sculpting on the journey to written reflection. This aligns with the idea of '*Presentational* knowing,' one of the four ways of knowing expounded by Heron and Reason (1997). It means creating knowledge based on our experiences (experiential knowing) through the medium of symbol, imagery and metaphor (presentational knowing) and feeds into our propositional knowing (knowing that…) and our practical knowing and action. Freya illustrates how presentational knowing enriches propositional knowing and articulation.

> I often struggle to put my feelings into words meaning my written reflections don't hold much tangible meaning for me. I find that the process of sculpting allows me to slow down and better explore complex feelings and the tactile sensation of sculpting allows for a calmer and less pressurised environment for reflection. As a result, sculpture allows me to articulate what I cannot with words. This can help me to eventually put my reflection into words as was the case with Growing Younger (see Figure 10.7). Below is the short reflection that I wrote after finishing the sculpture.

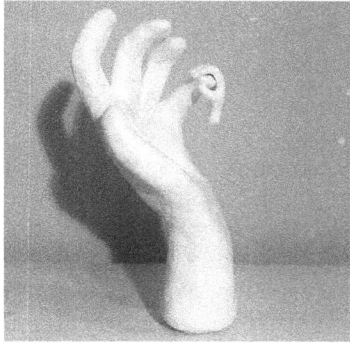

Figure 10.7 Growing Younger by Freya Qureshi (Qureshi, 2024).

For the earlier years of my degree, I often felt like an adult in a child's body, expected to mature at an exponential rate. Recently however I have begun to feel more like a small child in an adult's body. Transitioning from the comfort of familiar labs and lecture halls to the discomfort of unfamiliar corridors and vast wards has forced me to recognise my childlike naivety in these new settings. A transition can, nevertheless, be interpreted as a growth, and I do feel I am growing. I am learning. I am adapting. Like a child.

(Qureshi, 2024)

The arts can create a bridge of understanding

Connection with others in the small group creative enquiry sessions is always a theme in student small group reflections, being surprised about being able to 'open up and share with the group even though I barely knew them,' or 'how open and honest everyone [was],' and to hear that 'other students felt out of their depth.' Students describe learning from each other, and valuing each other:

I vividly recall being astounded at the support and warmth with which my peers approached my contribution… Many of us in the group noted through-out this SSC that our experience of medical school so far could often make us feel insignificant and unseen, but this SSC really gave us the chance to connect with each other and have our feelings heard.

(Younie & Adachi, 2024)

How might we introduce and facilitate creative enquiry?

To engage students, there is work to be done to find pedagogical approaches, language as well as facilitator development towards being able to enable creativity and hold transformative spaces. In a biomedically dominant paradigm, this work risks being dismissed as the 'soft stuff' (Younie, 2021a) and students can feel angry or exposed if clear framing for the purpose of the work and psychological safety are not established. Negative feedback over the years has been relatively limited by the fact that in the context of SSC, students have opted to engage with creativity. However, the kinds of student objections where this was made compulsory for all include: time could be better spent, no perceived benefit to career, confusion over assessment, cost of materials.

Easy ways to introduce creative enquiry include extending any written reflection, for example, on a clinical placement to include creative enquiry options. Students can be supported by 'show' rather than 'tell' approaches, offering examples from previous years or other courses, e.g. www.outofourheads.net and https://www.creativeenquiry.co.uk/artwork. Thought needs to go into how such creative-reflective assignments are assessed. We have created a framework drawing on ethnographic evaluation which often includes: perception, reflection, aesthetics and impact (Younie, 2011). Decisions need to be made regarding whether this is a formative or summative assignment. Often we have used a pass-fail summative approach because conversations around subjectivity in marking can become tricky with grades, but formative work may not be completed. A fail would be issued only where a student had made no reasonable attempt at the work. A way of insightful student work receiving wider audience is inviting nominations for a prize.

In the small group creative enquiry setting, creative exercises can lead to more personal sharing, e.g. choosing a postcard as illustrated above, or writing a Haiku, collaging, or taking photos. This is powerful, humanising and transformative but also has the potential to leave students feeling vulnerable or exposed. One student said on first sharing round the room of a creative doodle, that it is hard to share, as you cannot be creative without putting something of yourself in it. Figure 10.8 includes some considerations to bear in mind as facilitator.

Vulnerable leadership means sharing personal stories that enable others to share, carefully chosen to show it is safe to speak up in this space (Younie, 2016). Psychological safety is a concept pioneered by Amy Edmondson (Novartis Professor of Leadership and Management at the Harvard Business School), where teams are safe for interpersonal risk taking. This idea can be explicitly shared with participants (Edmondson et al., 2016). Equal voice comes from research at Google where they found the best teams are those where there is equal voice and social sensitivity across the group: the quality of the relationships is foundational (Duhigg, 2016). Moving on to boundaries, one way of creating safe boundaries is emerging a set of agreed group rules which hopefully include respect and confidentiality, and the valuing of diversity in thinking. In each creative exercise students are also invited to only share as much as they want to share, being able to talk about process rather than their actual creation if preferred.

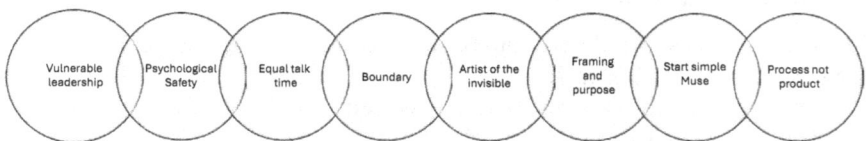

Figure 10.8 Facilitation Considerations (Younie, 2025).

Beyond these various strategies, there is an artistry to facilitation of transform-ative spaces. Seeley (2011) describes this as being 'artist of the invisible.' The facilitator needs to be reading the room, interpreting the dynamics and energy. It helps to be positioned as a co-learner as this enhances curiosity and allows ongoing and continual learning for this human-dimensions work. Artistry is also central to experimental introduction or crafting of creative exercises brought into land in a medical education context.

Framing the space and the purpose of the work are essential for student engage-ment. Modern agendas of 'managing uncertainty' or 'delivering person-centred care,' core tenets in the General Medical Council's MLA, are key areas where meaning making through creative enquiry can impact. To frame the space, I may highlight these areas. A particularly poignant introduction can be presenting and critiquing the idea of 'Medically Unexplained Symptoms,' proposing Launer's alternative of 'Medically Unexplored Stories' (Launer, 2009).

Starting with something simple that works as a creative muse is important in the light of students potentially feeling threatened, vulnerable or fearful about their level of artistic prowess. To help students adjust to a metaphorically rich learning environ-ment from the world of facts and skills, I slowly and gently encourage engagement with our metaphorical muscles, e.g. looking at what people see in an image on the screen, shared doodling, or collective poetry, e.g. where each person writes on a post-it to a prompt, e.g. 'I feel cared for when...' This can then be structured into a poem by the facilitator as their creative act during the session and shared at the end.

Participants are invited to move into process rather than product thinking, encouraging playful and improvisational engagement with materials which can take a while to sink in, but grow as the group relaxes into the creative enquiry space. We reassure them, we are not creating future professional artists but future doctors or practitioners who will find themselves in the complexity and messiness of clinical practice for which creativity, improvisation and artistry are essential.

All of these facilitation processes for enabling student engagement in creative enquiry are mirrored in faculty development, whether it be GP tutors wanting to know how to mark the emerging student creative-reflective work while on GP placement, or future creative enquiry facilitators wondering how to hold and create a safe space for this work or for postgraduate hospital and GP trainers wanting to develop their men-toring and supervision. Importantly, we engage the educators in the creative enquiry process, as the experience is better understood lived than talked about. In addition, we may consider the strengths and weaknesses pedagogically of these approaches, what are the challenges of facilitating these spaces and how to build flow and safety in the room as well as some of the different kinds of creative exercises that could be used.

The approaches described in this chapter, creative enquiry and Conversations Inviting Change have commonality. Both invite learners to use their creative agency to enhance meaning making and connection. In the case of CIC, practition-ers may help patients to find a different story; and in the process, may themselves re-discover a sense of meaning in their work. In the case of creative enquiry, stu-dents may end up understanding themselves better, including processing difficult emotions and making sense of the work they are being trained to do.

References

Anil, J., Cunningham, P., Dine, C. J., Swain, A., & DeLisser, H. M. (2023). The medical humanities at United States medical schools: A mixed method analysis of publicly assessable information on 31 schools. *BMC Medical Education, 23*(1), 620. https://doi.org/10.1186/s12909-023-04564-y

Bansal, A., Greenley, S., Mitchell, C., Park, S., Shearn, K., & Reeve, J. (2022). Optimising planned medical education strategies to develop learners' Person-Centredness: A realist review. *Medical Education, 56*(5), 489–503.

Banu, M. (2023). How may we learn about compassion? A pilot study. *Journal of Holistic Healthcare, 20*(2), 22–26.

Bovo, M. V., & Launer, J. (2022). 'Tell me about that colleague': Long COVID, narrative medicine, and a remarkable conversation. *British Journal of General Practice, 72*(719), 278–279.

Broyard, A. (1992). *Intoxicated by my illness: And other writings on life and death.* Fawcett.

Carel, H. (2008). *Illness: The cry of the flesh.* Routledge.

Charon, R. (2006). *Narrative medicine: Honoring the stories of illness.* Oxford University Press.

Czikszentmihalyi, M. (1990). *Flow: The psychology of optimal experience.* Harper & Row.

DasGupta, S. (2008). Narrative humility. *The Lancet, 371*(9617), 980–981.

Descouens, D. (2021). *The lady and the unicorn* (Photograph of tapestry in the Musée de Cluny). Wikimedia Commons. https://w.wiki/EZV8

Duhigg, C. (2016). What Google Learned from its Quest to Build the Perfect Team. *The New York Times Magazine.* https://www.nytimes.com/2016/02/28/magazine/what-google-learned-from-its-quest-to-build-the-perfect-team.html

Edmondson, A. C., Higgins, M., Singer, S., & Weiner, J. (2016). Understanding psychological safety in health care and education organizations: A comparative perspective. *Research in Human Development, 13*(1), 65–83.

Gadamer, H.- G. (1989). *Truth and method.* A&C Black.

Garaway, D. (2025). *A Barren Tree with Flowers Growing on the Roots* (Illustration). https://www.davidartlondon.co.uk/

Greenhalgh, T., & Hurwitz, B. (1998). *Narrative based medicine: Dialogue and discourse in clinical practice.* BMJ Books.

Guo, L. (2023). An overview of narrative medicine in China. *Chinese Medicine and Culture, 6*(2), 205–212.

Haidet, P. (2007). Jazz and the 'art' of medicine: Improvisation in the medical encounter. *The Annals of Family Medicine, 5*(2), 164–169.

Heron, J., & Reason, P. (1997). A participatory inquiry paradigm. *Qualitative Inquiry, 3*(3), 274–294.

Hicks, E. (2023). *Archaeologist excavating at Brimpton House.* Wikimedia Commons. https://commons.wikimedia.org/wiki/File:Archaeologist_excavation_at_Brimpton_House,_59A_High_Street,_Kelvedon,_Essex,_September_2023.jpg

Kinchin, I. M. (2023). Five moves towards an ecological university. *Teaching in Higher Education, 28*(5), 918–932.

Klem (2007). *Yin and yang symbol.* Wikimedia Commons. Labelling of figure by Dr Jens Foell. https://commons.wikimedia.org/wiki/File:Yin_and_Yang_symbol.svg

Kumagai, A. K. (2012). Perspective: Acts of interpretation: A philosophical approach to using creative arts in medical education. *Academic Medicine, 87*(8), 1138–1144.

Launer, J. (2009). Medically unexplored stories. *Postgraduate Medical Journal*, 85(1007), 503–504.

Launer, J. (2024). *Why is listening to a story more effective than "taking a history"?* https://www.conversationsinvitingchange.com/2024/06/07/why-is-listening-to-a-story-more-effective-than-taking-a-history/

Launer, J., & Lindsey, C. (1997). Training for systemic general practice: A new approach from the Tavistock Clinic. *British Journal of General Practice*, 47(420), 453–456.

Launer, J., & Wohlmann, A. (2023). Narrative medicine, narrative practice, and the creation of meaning. *The Lancet*, 401(10371), 98–99. https://doi.org/10.1016/s0140-6736(23)00017-x

Mandourah, S. (2024). The cracks. *Journal of Holistic Healthcare*, 21(1), 17.

Milligan, E., & Woodley, E. (2009). Creative expressive encounters in health ethics education: Teaching ethics as relational engagement. *Teaching and Learning in Medicine*, 21(2), 131–139.

Polkinghorne, D. E. (1988). *Narrative knowing and the human sciences*. SUNY Press.

Qureshi, F. (2024). Growing younger: Sculpture as a form of reflection. *Journal of Holistic Healthcare*, 21(1), 18.

Reeve, J. (2017). Unlocking the creative capacity of the self. In *Person-centred primary care* (pp. 141–165). Routledge.

Seeley, C. (2011). Uncharted territory: Imagining a stronger relationship between the arts and action research. *Action Research*, 9(1), 83–99.

Shah, R., Clarke, R., Ahluwalia, S., & Launer, J. (2020). Finding meaning in the consultation: introducing the hermeneutic window. *British Journal of General Practice*, 70(699), 502–503.

Shapiro, J. (2009). *The inner world of medical students listening to their voices in poetry*. Radcliffe Publishing.

White, M., & and Epston, D. (1990). *Narrative means to therapeutic ends*. Norton.

Younie, L. (2006). *A qualitative study of the contribution medical humanities can bring to medical education*. University of Bristol.

Younie, L. (2009). Developing narrative competence in medical students. *Medical humanities*, 35(1), 54–54.

Younie, L. (2011). *A reflexive journey through arts-based inquiry in medical education* University of Bristol.

Younie, L. (2013). Introducing arts-based inquiry into medical education: 'Exploring the creative arts in health and illness'. In P. McIntosh & D. Warren (Eds.), *Creativity in the classroom: Case studies in using the arts in teaching and learning in higher education* (pp. 23–40). Intellect Publishers.

Younie, L. (2014). Arts-based inquiry and a clinician educator's journey of discovery. In C. L. McLean (Eds.), *Creative arts in humane medicine* (pp. 163–180). Brush Education Inc.

Younie, L. (2016). Vulnerable leadership. *London Journal of Primary Care*, 8(3), 37–38. https://doi.org/10.1080/17571472.2016.1163939

Younie, L. (2019a). *Flourishing through creative enquiry.* Retrieved 29/12/2024 from https://sites.google.com/view/humanflourishingmeded/creative-enquiry-projects/creative-arts-ssc

Younie, L. (2019b). Vulnerability, resilience and the arts. In J. K. Patterson, & F. Kinchington (Eds.), *Body talk: Whose language* (pp. 64–77). Cambridge Scholars Publishing.

Younie, L. (2021). What does creative enquiry have to contribute to flourishing in medical education? In E. B. Murray, J. (Ed.), *The mental health and wellbeing of healthcare practitioners: Research and practice* (pp. 14–27). Wiley-Blackwell.

Younie, L. (2021a). Humanising medical education. *Journal of Holistic Healthcare, 18,* 37–39.

Younie, L. (2022). Compassion–walking the walk, who does the talk? *Journal of Holistic Healthcare and Integrative Medicine, 19*(3), 31.

Younie, L. (2025). *Facilitation considerations* (Unpublished diagram).

Younie, L., & Adachi, C. (2024). Nurturing the human dimension in digital and medical spaces through pedagogy of care – A case of creative enquiry. *Perspectives on Medical Education, 13*(1), 307–312. https://doi.org/10.5334/pme.1147

11 A hermeneutic approach to professionalism and the link with practical wisdom

Sabena Jameel

In a world increasingly driven by rationalism and measurable outcomes, where is the space for engaging in interpretative processes and making meaning of what we do? In medicine, the structures of education and practice have marginalised these opportunities. This chapter outlines my observations on the current situation, explores the reasons behind these trends, and proposes a way forward.

I will present a couple of dilemmas I have contemplated, informed by my experience as an inner-city general practitioner and as a senior medical educator working in both postgraduate and undergraduate settings. The most exciting aspect of this exploration is translating the ideas from my doctoral thesis on practical wisdom and professionalism into a form that clinicians can readily understand. Meaning is rooted in understanding.

Throughout my journey, I have tried hard to articulate what many of my peers and colleagues have felt but lacked the language to express. This is a synthesis of what I have observed. My aim is to foster a deeper understanding of our practice.

Dilemma 1: finding the right language

Words are complicated and rarely express what you mean; not because feelings cannot be explained with words, but the moment that we start choosing words to explain ourselves, our feelings are no longer the same.

Jeanette Ringel

In the early days of my PhD, I remember sitting in an academic seminar on the philosophy of research. The erudite professor was using terms which alienated me, 'blah blah blah *ontology* and *epistemology*.' I felt dazed and dumbfounded. He seemed so au-fait with the terms and I could grasp neither their meaning, nor their application. I felt very stupid and disempowered. That feeling, to this day, keeps me humble and mindful. My thesis examined phronesis in medicine, phronesis being an ancient Greek term for practical wisdom. I needed to navigate a path which persuaded busy clinicians that these ideas are still relevant, rather than making them feel alienated and uninterested. I had done some background reading on phronesis, so I knew it had resonance with the work of clinicians. It was in the early

DOI: 10.4324/9781003517665-11

1990s when the term phronesis was revived (post-Aristotle) and purported to be highly relevant to the work of a doctor (Pellegrino & Thomasma, 1993), but there was little empirical research. I felt passionate that it was a term that would add value and help us understand our role better, even though it was almost 3,000 years old. So, my first dilemma was in communicating that concept. I wanted closeness, not distance.

When I pondered over the choice of phronesis, the Ringel quote above seemed very relevant (Ringel, 2017). We may not have words that express what we feel, but if we use a proxy, does that change what we feel? There is interesting work on different languages, neuroprocessing and meaning in relation to how we see the world. I felt phronesis was worthy of exploration; it introduced a virtue literacy term that had been buried in the rise of positivistic approaches to medicine and medical education that sideline values, opinions and feelings in the quest to be objective and value-free.

It is evident that the term *Hermeneutics* has a similar effect, with a small survey of trainees and GPs showing that 20% do not have the time for it and 20% do not even understand the concept when asked during a series of workshops run by Rupal Shah (personal communication, 2024). At its core, hermeneutics is about interpretation and making meaning, which has undoubted importance in navigating life. In relation to the GP consultation, Shah et al write:

> The hermeneutic window is where assumptions, meanings, and roles are interpreted in a way particular to the patient, doctor, and circumstances, and to the moment. This is often the area of greatest complexity and uncertainty, where questions about what it means to be a healthcare professional are asked and relationships with individual patients are examined.
>
> (Shah et al., 2021)

Compare this to quotes on practical wisdom in medicine, with the second being my conclusion after my empirical work was completed:

> Physicians need wisdom in medical decision making because of the nature of human beings and the illness they experience. The landscape of medicine entails complexity, uncertainty, fluidity, particularity, morality, and diversity. Not to mention the technological questions and therapeutic options.
>
> (Kaldjian, 2019)

> A practically wise doctor does the right thing, at the right time for the right reason (morally orientated) in context. A practically wise doctor can adjudicate when values conflict, thus is comfortable in dealing with uncertainty; they aspire to make an all-things-considered judgement. They are self-aware, reflective and secure in their professional identity.
>
> (Jameel, 2021)

Practitioner as witness	Intuition in partnership with evidence
Practitioner's biographical function	How do I sense this?
Practitioner's use of self	How do I use the different ways of knowing?

Hermeneutic window

Narrative practice	Exploring professionalism
Emotional engagement and connection	What is my role here?
Authenticity and curiosity	What assumptions am I making?
Relational ethical framework	How do my own experiences affect the interaction?

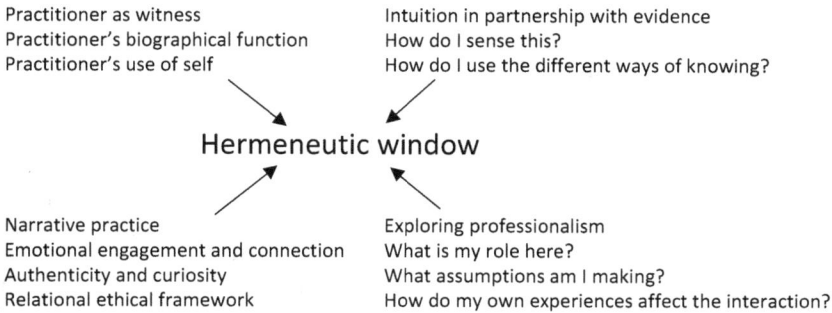

Figure 11.1 Opening Up the Hermeneutic Window (Shah et al., 2021).

Can we therefore assert that educating for phronesis/practical wisdom enables clinicians to work more comfortably in the hermeneutic window? I think that is not unreasonable, and that is where this chapter comes together. See Figure 11.1.

So, what has this got to do with professionalism? Everyone knows what professionalism means don't they? Well, no! In 2020 I became medical professionalism lead at a large UK medical school. I was tasked with devising a new professionalism curriculum across all five years. It became clear that there was no consensus definition of professionalism and the predominant understanding was formed around professionalism in relation to General Medical Council and UK legal obligations. There was a sense of disempowerment, with some colleagues referring to the GMC as the mafia or the clergy, telling them what to do to be professional.

In response, the very first series of lectures I delivered was entitled 'How to make professionalism work for you.' I was able to reclaim professionalism as being as much to do with character development and professional identity as it was to do with the regulatory aspects. This aligned with the work of Irby and Hamstra who wrote a paper entitled, 'Parting the clouds' where they described the behaviour-based, virtue-based and identity formation aspects of educating for medical professionalism (Irby & Hamstra, 2016). I have continued to favour a few key definitions of professionalism; these reinforce its expansive nature, with my overarching curriculum being known as 'Radial Holistic Professionalism.' I emphasise that professionalism is a *trust-generating promise* (Brody & Doukas, 2014) and present professionalism as the *morality of medicine* (Bontemps-Hommen et al., 2019), along with a longer definition from a systematic review by Ong et al. (2020), which helps students understand the evolving nature of professionalism and four key areas of professional development.

What all this really enabled me to do was to translate some ideas from my doctorate work to tangibly influence students, who are the future of medicine. It enabled me to shift to a wisdom approach in medical education. This was inspired by a synergy that Kinghorn suggested when he proposed that phronesis aligns with the modern conceptualisation of professionalism (Kinghorn, 2010).

In summary, to tackle dilemma 1, the unfamiliar term *phronesis* becomes embedded in the more familiar term *professionalism,* which, in turn, can help us to enter the *hermeneutic window.*

Dilemma 2: persuading boiling frogs to jump out of the saucepan

Fables are a time-old tradition that use storytelling narrative to convey an important moral lesson. At the outset they may seem the antithesis of scientific method, yet they are still an impactful way to impart knowledge, wisdom and understanding. Making meaning is a moral act that shapes our beliefs, values and actions. The process of interpreting and understanding our experiences (hermeneutics) carries ethical significance, especially in medicine. It can influence our decisions, relationships, and contributions to society.

Have you heard of the fable describing a frog being slowly boiled alive? The story is a metaphor for our inability to react to insidious threat. If you put a frog in hot water, it will immediately jump out, but if you put a frog in tepid water and slowly bring it to boil, the frog won't sense the threat and will fail to resist its demise. Allow me to suggest that we are those frogs in the warming water, unaware of the climate that erodes our moral development as healthcare practitioners.

In this section I will outline historic (and maintained) structural and organisational norms that have served important purposes, but that have been deficient in attending to morals and values. In this way, they have inadvertently contributed to the demoralisation of the healthcare workforce, whose members notice that their values no longer align with the demands made of them. I will refer to the ethical frameworks that underpin healthcare, then move to the educational frameworks and tools that are in common use. I then suggest that my next big dilemma lies in how to introduce new ways of thinking, like a wisdom approach to medical education, that do not easily fit into current organisational and educational structures. Catalysing change is a huge undertaking because 'the establishment' likes the status quo.

The predominant ethical frameworks that shape healthcare are essentially all rules-based or code-based, outside-in frameworks. This means they are a set of externally determined, generalisable rules that clinicians are expected to apply unquestioningly to any context. Good Medical Practice (GMC, 2024) is based on Kant's deontological ideas. The formation of the National Health Service (NHS) is rooted in Utilitarian-Consequentialist concepts (Bentham and Mill), with the health of the nation being the single currency outcome. More recently with healthcare commissioning, free commercial markets have become normalised and this is considered libertarian (described by William Belsham in 1789). All these paradigms have shortcomings, particularly when their use is advocated in the complex, messy, relational world of healthcare: for example, in the context of safeguarding, decisions about capacity and mental health.

Schwartz and Sharp argue that rules fail; and further, that rules undermine skill; and that incentives undermine will. Thus, the tools that organisations commonly use to control and regulate are counter-productive (Schwartz & Sharpe, 2010). This differentiation has been nicely illustrated in a nursery experiment, which imposed a monetary fine for late collection of children. Prior to the fine, parents would show remorse to staff if they arrived late. Implementing the fine did not achieve the stated goal of getting staff home on time; in fact more parents chose to come late, accepting the fine. On removing the penalty, collection behaviour did not improve and remorse was no longer a feature, thus suggesting that effective methods of change should encompass moral, social and economic incentives (Gneezy & Rustichini, 2000). The lessons from this experiment can be extrapolated to help us understand clinicians' behaviour in a context where there is a rule for every eventuality. This is, of course, very relevant when considering professionalism in relation to phronesis.

Don Berwick, a former healthcare advisor to the Obama administration, and Kings Fund, international visiting fellow, wrote a sagacious short paper on three eras of healthcare. In this he explains that era 1 was the *Ascendency era*, where medical idealism and high trust was marred by variations in practice, abuse of privilege and inequalities. This led to era 2, the *Protectionist era*, which we currently inhabit. It is an era of scrutiny, accountability and bureaucracy (Berwick, 2016). It has paved the way for incentives, performance related pay and punishment. Inspection, control, and regulation are the new norms, seemingly in order to demonstrate accountability to service users (patients). The meaning of service has changed rapidly, from the rather altruistic notion of serving someone out of duty and humility, to a system predicated around supplying a consumer. With this consumerism has come a shift in language. Patients are now service users, who are entitled to receive health services but who are owed no moral duty by their clinicians, transforming the clinical encounter from interaction to transaction. Medicine has become industrialised (Montori, 2020).

Phronesis is an intellectual virtue that sits in an alternative ethical framework, *virtue ethics*. It is inherently 'unruly' for organisations that depend on certainty of outcomes and control. Virtue ethics is an inside-out framework that seeks to find out what it means to live (or practise) well, with character education being core to this goal. These concepts are hard to measure and difficult to audit. The moral pluralism, subjectivity and lack of clear guidance make it difficult to implement with any consistency. It is not favoured by organisations. The irony is that we expect clinicians to be competent at dealing with uncertainty, but they must work in systems where certainty and accountability are the only way, with little flexibility.

Another deeply embedded way-of-doing-things are the educational frameworks that shape medical education. I refer to four main frameworks outlined by Illing: positivism, post-positivism, critical theory and constructivism (Illing, 2007). Empiricism, technical rationality and certainty were hailed as the nation's saviours in the age of enlightenment, influenced significantly by Descartes (1637 AD). These positivist ideas align very well with latter developments in medical education, led by Abraham Flexner (1910). Scientific method and positivistic ways of obtaining evidence based knowledge have meant we have enjoyed incredible advances in medicine, but this has come at the expense of neglecting other ways of knowing; sidelining constructivism and critical theory. It is these frameworks that enable and promote conversations about values, opinion and feelings, all essential for medical hermeneutics and for professionalism.

Berwick observes this is where the romance of autonomy in era 1 clashes with the external accountability of era 2. Many doctors have become disillusioned, so he proposes an era 3, the moral era:

When the ethos of professionalism clashes with the ethos of markets and accountability, immense resources get diverted from the crucial and difficult enterprise of recreating care.

(Berwick, 2016)

Berwick outlines nine necessary changes in medicine and healthcare in working towards the third era – the *Moral era*:

1 Stop excessive measurement.
2 Abandon complex incentives.
3 Reduce the focus on finance but increase attention to quality of care.
4 Reduce professional prerogative.
5 Recommit to improvement science.
6 Embrace transparency.
7 Protect civility.
8 Really listen (especially to the poor, disadvantaged and excluded).
9 Reject greed (it erodes trust).

Eight years on, have we digested and acted on these wise recommendations? I am not sure we have, because large scale change is difficult, and *the large tanker is slow to turn*, with momentum maintaining the status quo.

I wrote earlier about my efforts to devise a new professionalism curriculum, the delivery of which was going well until I was asked to use Blooms Taxonomy to specify the skills and knowledge I expected students to acquire and to describe my intended learning outcomes. Although it is so deeply embedded in our educational paradigm that questioning it feels heretical, I found Bloom's cognitive taxonomy (1956) to be a deficient model when considering professionalism. Professionalism involves BEING as well as DOING. BEING is difficult to assess. Bloom's taxonomy was later refined to include lesser-known affective levels and psychomotor levels (Bloom, 1982). These are more useful in considering the emotional regulation and the invention required in developing professional identity, but are hardly ever adopted in educational systems.

When I explain to my learners that the education system is biased and that the ethical frameworks that shape healthcare are deficient, they begin to realise that what is missing is the *moral mode of practice*. The frameworks that enable us to make meaning by exploring values and feelings, have been removed from our widely adopted systems. It then becomes clear why we are demoralised, because there is no real room for morality.

Do we accept this status quo? No. By collaborative works such as this book, by raising awareness of the rising water temperature and by calling for meaningful change towards moral and humane practice, I believe we can address the imbalances and draw upon those unique, 'complicated' words that have special meaning; phronesis and hermeneutics, to understand the world better and improve medical education and professionalism in practice

References

Belsham, W. (1789). *Essays, philosophical, historical, and literary* (Vol. 1). C. Dilly.

Berwick, D. M. (2016). Era 3 for medicine and health care. *Journal of the American Medical Association, 315*(13), 1329–1330.

Bloom, B. S. (1982). The role of gifts and markers in the development of talent. *Exceptional Children, 48*(6), 510–522. https://doi.org/10.1177/001440298204800607

Bontemps-Hommen, C., Baart, A., & Vosman, F. T. H. (2019). Practical wisdom in complex medical practices: A critical proposal. *Medical Health Care and Philosophy, 22*(1), 95–105. https://doi.org/10.1007/s11019-018-9846-x

Brody, H., & Doukas, D. (2014). Professionalism: A framework to guide medical education. *Medical Education, 48*(10), 980–987. https://doi.org/10.1111/medu.12520

Flexner, A. (1910). *Medical education in the United States and Canada: A report to the Carnegie Foundation for the advancement of teaching.* Carnegie Foundation for the Advancement of Teaching.

GMC. (2024). *Good medical practice.* Retrieved 13/06/2024 from https://www.gmc-uk.org/professional-standards/good-medical-practice-2024

Gneezy, U., & Rustichini, A. (2000). A fine is a price. *The Journal of Legal Studies, 29*(1), 1–17. https://doi.org/10.1086/468061

Irby, D. M., & Hamstra, S. J. (2016). Parting the clouds: Three professionalism frameworks in medical education. *Academic Medicine, 91*(12), 1606–1611.

Jameel, S. (2021). *Enacted phronesis in general practitioners.* University of Birmingham. https://etheses.bham.ac.uk/id/eprint/12197/

Kaldjian, L. C. (2019). Wisdom in medical decision-making. In R. J. Sternberg & J. Glück (Eds.), *The Cambridge handbook of wisdom.* Cambridge University Press.

Kinghorn, W. A. (2010). Medical education as moral formation: An Aristotelian account of medical professionalism. *Perspectives in Biology and Medicine, 53*(1), 87–105.

Montori, V. (2020). *Why we revolt: A patient revolution for careful and kind care.* Rosetta Books.

Ong, Y. T., Kow, C. S., Teo, Y. H., Tan, L. H. E., Abdurrahman, A. B. H. M., Quek, N. W. S., Prakash, K., Cheong, C. W. S., Tan, X. H., & Lim, W. Q. (2020). Nurturing professionalism in medical schools. A systematic scoping review of training curricula between 1990–2019. *Medical Teacher, 42*(6), 636–649.

Pellegrino, E. D., & Thomasma, D. (1993). *The virtues in medical practice* (Vol. 86). Oxford University Press.

Ringel, J. (2017). Sea of clouds. Createspace.

Schwartz, B., & Sharpe, K. (2010). *Practical Wisdom: The right way to do the right thing by.* Riverhead books.

Shah, R., Clarke, R., Ahluwalia, S., & Launer, J. (2021). Finding meaning in the consultation: Working in the hermeneutic window. *British Journal of General Practice, 71*(707), 282–283.

12 Flourishing spaces

Louise Younie

Medicine is founded upon an explicit biomedical curriculum which prioritises science over relationship (Heath, 2018) and has a hidden curriculum shaped by macho invulnerability (Cribb & Bignold, 1999). Yet there is a growing 'wellness crisis' amongst students and clinicians (BMA, 2019; West & Coia, 2019) which is risky for clinicians themselves, and also the patients they serve (Panagioti et al., 2018; Shanafelt et al., 2010). Whilst the research is clear that we face an epidemic of burnout, moral injury and impaired mental health in medical students and doctors (Asta et al., 2023; Hartzband & Groopman, 2020), what is less clear is what to do about it (Dyrbye et al., 2005). One approach which gained traction over the last 20 years has been a focus on building and developing resilience in our future clinicians: articles documented on PubMed relating to 'resilience in healthcare' increased from 38 in 2004 to 1842 in November 2024. Increasingly, the way in which resilience training has been wielded against beleaguered and burnt out students and colleagues has been critiqued, by myself (Younie, 2019, 2020) and others (Card, 2018; Taylor, 2019) and most amusingly by Glaukomflecken in his YouTube skit where he plays both weary doctor and officious manager (Glaucomflecken, 2022).

Alongside a variety of colleagues and teams, I have been seeking to move the conversation in higher education and healthcare from resilience towards human flourishing, creating a different kind of space to consider our humanity in the face of the systems we serve. We are not so interested in measuring flourishing, as, for example, is being done by The Human Flourishing Programme at Harvard (VanderWeele, 2017), but instead consider how we may grow and move towards flourishing. This has led to greater interest not just in our own individual flourishing and what that actually means, but we seek to better understand the attributes of study and workspaces that enable flourishing. To this end we are conducting research, exploring practice and developing collaborations under the banner of 'Flourishing Spaces.' We cannot do this, however, without recognising the challenges we face. In this chapter, I will explore some of these, specifically the impact of neoliberalism, of parched relationships and connections, including with ourselves and how resilience training may not be helping. Subsequently I consider what flourishing might look like in practice and how we might create, enable or find flourishing spaces.

DOI: 10.4324/9781003517665-12

The neoliberal desert

Neoliberalism is an outlook or approach founded in the 1930s in Europe and translated and propagated at the University of Chicago by names like Hayek, Knight, Friedman and Stigler (Metcalf, 2017; Monbiot, 2016). They went on to establish the Chicago School of Economics, which later influenced US and UK politics (Fisher, 2007).

The focus of neoliberalism is on market efficiency, individualism and competition, with humans redefined as 'consumers' in 'the market' rather than 'bearers of grace' or having 'inalienable rights and duties' (Metcalf, 2017). In this worldview, previously non-economic domains become reinterpreted in terms of market metrics, penetrating into, for example, the educational, political and cultural spheres (Brown, 2015) and seeming to imply a machine model of healthcare, where human experience is sidelined.

The neoliberal agenda is clear – deregulation on economies, opening national markets to trade, lowering taxes and privatising the public sphere (Klein, 2007). Neoliberalism is a set of lenses through which to see the world (Metcalf, 2017), where the human creature is marked down as essentially selfish and with competition the only way to regulate what we practise and believe (Metcalf, 2017). In this world view the human is translated into homo economicus (Brown, 2015).

In the healthcare setting, the neoliberal competitive agenda focusses on measurable outcomes such as productivity, profit, performance metrics, inevitably sidelining the human dimension of clinical practice such as meaning making, human connection, quality of relationship, trust, feeling listened to, as well as the time for clinician self-reflection and growth – much of what we have described as being within the hermeneutic window. Consultations are curtailed by lack of time, the need to meet quotas and institutional demands, stripping away space for compassion and meaning making. Of course, we still encounter many empathic clinicians but as Hartzman puts it in a paper entitled 'Physician Burnout Interrupted' (Hartzband & Groopman, 2020):

> Physicians recognize that it's impossible to satisfy the current system's demands. If you surrender, the joy of engaging with your patients is diminished and ultimately lost. If you resist, you incur the system's wrath.

The system's wrath may mean running very late, a heavier emotional workload, engaging increasingly with suffering and trauma without adequate support and infrastructure, not being heard or valued by the system due to slower practice, etc. Hartzman, writing from a US perspective goes on to say (Hartzband & Groopman, 2020):

> Doctors want to give patients the time and support they need, and they want the system to value and recognize their efforts to provide this kind of care. While much lip service is given to "patient centered care," many doctors feel that the system is increasingly driven by money and metrics, with rewards for professionals who embrace these priorities.

This is compounded by biomedicine where the foundational building block is the randomised double blind controlled trial. Of course, so much has been won in medical practice through randomised controlled trials. What is lost is the idea that clinicians themselves have anything more to bring than a subjective placebo effect to be edited out of these studies. Here biomedicine as 'scientific' and 'objective' partnered with a neoliberal market economy view, powerfully intersect to create a heady mixture where the humanity of the clinician is so devalued that clinicians and students themselves buy into this narrative.

> Physicians have lost confidence in themselves. They no longer consider it professional to help patients by their words, by their person, or by their presence.
>
> (Spiro, 2004)

Resilience – a neoliberal concept?

Within this context of the struggling or even missing (in their humanity) healthcare professional/clinician, the concept of resilience may add insult to injury. Resilience has been held up as a panacea for our 'wellness crisis' in medicine (Teodorczuk et al., 2017), typically framed as an individual capacity for positivity and 'bouncing back' in adversity. The Latin root is 'resilire' to 'spring back' or 'rebound.' In the physical sciences, resilience indicates materials resuming their original shape after being bent or stretched. Translated to humans, this suggests withstanding challenges and an individual capacity to be tough and unchanged through adversity (Van der Kolk, 2014). In this way, it could be argued that resilience aligns with the neoliberal agenda in that individuals are responsible for their own social and economic security and that states or institutions bear no collective responsibility. Those who are struggling become 'deficient subjects unable to adjust to the requirements of modern life' (Mavelli, 2019) with burnout understood to be the result of being a 'weak' individual (Van der Kolk, 2014).

Resilience may make sense within the neoliberal machine: try harder, give more, compete and win. However, there is extensive criticism of resilience in the literature. This ranges from concluding that resilience training is '*only part of the solution*' (Card, 2018), i.e. only useful to support capacity for unavoidable challenges such as repeated encountering of patient suffering and not for avoidable organisation-based issues (Card, 2018); to at the other end, recognising 'resilience shaming' of clinicians with their tendency to perfectionism and self-blame and even arguing that resilience can be 'abusive' or 'damaging' when focussed purely on the individual and not the environment. Research has in fact found that the high burnout rate in doctors is not due to deficiency in resilience, doctors having higher than average resilience scores (West et al., 2020) and 29% of physicians with the highest possible resilience score were still found to be experiencing burnout (West et al., 2020). Resilience training in healthcare professionals has been likened to making the canary we send down the mine stronger to survive the toxicity of the mine (Sinskey et al., 2022).

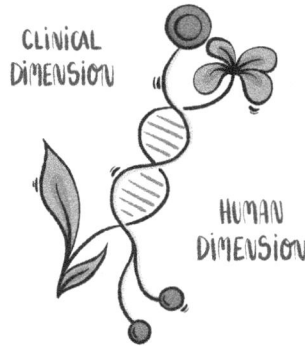

Figure 12.1 Clinical and Human Dimensions © Camille Aubry, Used with Permission (Aubry, 2025).

Seeking to challenge the trend away from humanity in healthcare means pitting ourselves in an 'uphill battle' (Tilburt & Geller, 2007). There is less credence than deserved for the human dimension, illustrated, for example, by denigrating the human dimension as the 'soft stuff' (Dowrick et al., 2016). Testimonial injustice, i.e. deflating someone's credibility (Fricker, 2007) can be the result of seeking to give voice to the importance of the human and relational for patient outcomes. There is also hermeneutic injustice due to the gap in shared tools of social interpretation (Fricker, 2007), seen in the challenge of finding shared language for teaching on, examining and explaining the human dimension. Expression of lived experience, verbalising what is complex, messy, often unseen and not easily measurable is difficult in a world where numbers and facts count.

To summarise this section: in the neoliberal paradigm, the clinician and patient are considered in relation to their market value, the 'homo economicus' and in biomedicine, a placebo effect to be ruled out so we can see the real effect of the drug or intervention. Testimonial and hermeneutic injustice compound the challenge of recognising, promoting, researching or voicing the value of the human dimension for the patient or the doctor alike. Trying to rectify the situation by offering the struggling healthcare professional resiliency modules that are framed within the idea of clinician deficiency feels like the wrong solution to the wrong problem. As Einstein said, 'We cannot solve our problems with the same thinking we used when we created them.'

As introduction to the next section, Figure 12.1 commissioned from @CamilleAubry casts a vision for the *human dimension* as part of the double stranded DNA of our consultations or our healthcare education alongside the *clinical dimension* (Younie, 2021b).

Flourishing

Neoliberalism offers one specific lens through which to view the world and ourselves within it. Flourishing offers us another set of lenses, valuing the human being as innately of precious worth. Perhaps if we were to realise that the greatest resource in healthcare is the people working in it, such an approach might even make economic sense in the end given the vast sums of money it costs to train clinicians and the cost of sick leave and attrition from the work force (Hartzband & Groopman, 2020). Here, I will argue for a move away from a scarcity towards an abundance mindset, from a zero-sum fearful approach where there is a finite pie of resources (time, money, opportunities), towards the idea that resources can be shared and even multiplied through collaborative regenerative approaches (Ichioka & Pawlyn, 2021). For example, this might include building trust in an organisation and enhancing collaboration or when an individual consultation involves a patient and clinician meaningfully connecting in a way that nourishes both.

The draw of human flourishing

For over 20 years, I have been exploring creative enquiry in medical education and beyond with the aim of promoting person-centred care and human flourishing. Perhaps it is the creative dimension that is particular in this work. Creative enquiry is the exploring of lived experience through any of the arts and it can be transformative and reach parts that other educational approaches cannot, especially in the field of the human dimension (Brown & Younie, 2022; Younie, 2021b). This is an example of a student creative enquiry piece produced as an end product on a two-week optional Student Selected Component.

The ups and downs of being a medical student by Benita (2018)

A theme that arose was that of the doctor's humanity coupling 'unrealistic expectations' with 'human' and similarly 'losing individuality' with 'the rawness of life and death'. Often, doctors are seen not to be human. They are expected to conform to a system and meet robotic unrealistic standards. At the same time, I realised that on the contrary a doctor is present at a patient's most vulnerable and pivotal moments and that the constant face of suffering helps one understand what it truly means to be human.

Creative enquiry allows the voicing of lived experience and connection with the messiness and complexity of our work. I discovered, that as we humanised patients (important in person-centred care (Bansal et al., 2022), doctors also became humanised and slowly I saw a different kind of wellbeing emerge: a wellbeing that was interpersonal, compassionate and connected, that engaged with the reality of clinical practice as it is, rather than an idealised and imagined doctor-patient scenario. What Creative Enquiry offers beyond more traditional educational approaches is listening with our own ears and seeing with our own eyes. Creative enquiry invites story-telling and expression that is multilingual, through the metaphors and symbolism of arts-based languages, in addition to written reflective prose (Younie, 2021a). The creative enquiry process, alongside vulnerable leadership (Younie, 2016) and transformative facilitation (Younie, 2014) catalyses expression and engagement with the contours of lived experience (Younie, 2021c). As we share lived experience through our creations, this can enable us to more fully connect with ourselves, each other and with meaning making in our work. These are all dimensions of human flourishing and opposite to the alienation that Gabor Mate describes in a video on 'why you feel so lost today' (Mate, 2019). We are alienated from ourselves, from each other, from meaningful work and from the environment, he says. One approach I take to explaining flourishing is to argue that flourishing is the connection in each of those areas.

What is flourishing?

Human flourishing is an old but new concept. Flourishing is old, in that Aristotle's eudaimonia, which was originally translated as happiness, has now latterly been described as flourishing. It is used to denote that part of wellbeing that relates to meaning and purpose, complementing hedonia: engaging with pleasurable activities for a quick fix, e.g. eating chocolate, or buying a new car (Huta, 2015). Flourishing is also new. There is now burgeoning engagement in what flourishing might mean or contribute in scholarly, clinical and policy spheres (Willen et al., 2022). Examples include the Templeton Foundation, which is investing $100 million into flourishing research, practices, and policies and the Kern National Network for Flourishing in Medicine, a national US-based movement seeking to catalyse transformative initiatives and influence policy and systems change. There is also the Human Flourishing Programme at Harvard which is well recognised globally. However, flourishing in healthcare education is not found much in the literature, with papers on resilience in healthcare ten-fold more common on PubMed to date. Examples in medical education that were found include themes of flourishing and trauma-informed care (Whitaker et al., 2024), flourishing in the clerkship year (Flickinger et al., 2022) and flourishing drawing on positive psychology (Slavin et al., 2011).

The term flourishing is not universal or clearly defined in healthcare and medicine (Levin, 2021). I have been seeking over many years, to develop a sharable useful conceptualisation of flourishing. I have used the online tool menti to create word clouds, asking participants to add one word that speaks to them of human flourishing. Often, we end up with 'growth' or 'blossom' larger and in the centre, highlighting that two or three people have chosen this word, and perhaps connecting with metaphorical significance of the word. The word flourish comes from the Latin *florere* 'to bloom, blossom, flower.'

An example word cloud from a Human Values in Healthcare conference in 2024 is shown in Figure 12.2, based on the question 'In one word what does flourishing mean to you?'

I learn from all the groups that I take these ideas out to. In one session with a non-medical audience, a participant asked, 'if you are happy but not growing are you flourishing?'. I bring this as a rhetorical question to other groups that I facilitate on the subject. Students, in particular, process the ideas that I share in their groups and then often share back new ideas to extend thinking in the field, in the form of creative expression or written prose. One student described flourishing as

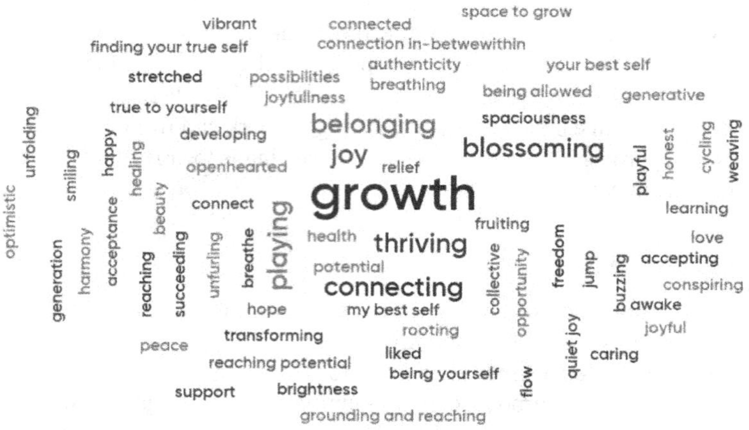

Figure 12.2 Flourishing Wordcloud (Younie, 2024).

a kinder way to grow, a state that did not require her to bounce back as if she had permanent springs under her shoes:

> I don't have to bounce back from every hard experience like I had permanent springs under my shoes- they are not permanent and they get rusty easily. The journey towards flourishing allows me to take painful experiences with me, explore them through creative enquiry, and accept them as part of me rather than as flaws I would like to exclude from my life.
>
> Elle Tallgren, 2022

Two other medical students captured some of what I offered on resilience and flourishing repackaging it through their own poetry in a creative writing session (see Figure 12.3).

I often end sessions by asking 'what stood out today?', and sometimes, 'what questions remain?'. Here are two example responses from Postgraduate GP Specialty Training Scheme participants in 2023.

> The whole concept of flourishing because it was the first time I ever heard about it being connected to medicine
> A new mindset: you don't need to suffer/stretch and bounce back: you can include the experiences and grow as a person.

Human flourishing models

A number of models exist to convey flourishing, e.g. Keyes' measurable scale from flourishing to languishing (Keyes, 2002), Seligman's PERMA (positive emotion, engagement, relationship, meaning and achievement) model (Seligman, 2011) and VanderWeele's six-domain scale, including numerically

Resilience

R eally push yourself to limits

E xcel in everything you do

S top letting hardships affect you

I nvest in yourself

L eave nothing to chance

I t is no big deal

E xpect greatness

N o matter the

C ircumstances

E verything always

By Grace Boyle

Flourish

F inding yourself

L iving with mistakes

O pening yourself to new experiences

U nderstanding it's OK to change

R ealising growth is not linear

I nviting forgiveness

S taying true

H olding space

By Naimaah Ahmed

Figure 12.3 Acrostic Poems on Resilience and Flourishing (Unpublished Work).

assessing our financial stability or our physical and mental health (VanderWeele, 2017). They all include relationship and meaning making (Willen et al., 2022), two elements that also feature in my own flourishing model which has emerged through creative enquiry practice with medical students. However, in my model (Younie, 2023, 2024) I also include 'shadow work,' a concept highlighted by Jung and which I simply take to mean engaging with the difficult stuff in us or in our lives (Jung, 2014). It is not necessarily an obvious part of flourishing, but I would argue that it is the most important part, because suffering is part of life and we all struggle in our different ways. Figure 12.4 illustrates five components of flourishing: ecological, making connections, meaning making, compassion and shadow work.

Finding spaces where this can be given voice builds community and rehumanises us in the face of our own potential critical or fearful judgement. I call this the wellbeing of 'what is' or 'what is found there' (Scannell, 2002) rather than 'try harder' simplistic messages of 'eat well,' 'sleep well,' 'exercise,' as valuable as those things are.

Theoretical underpinning: self-determination theory

Neoliberalism has been found to reduce individual wellbeing by promoting social disconnection, competition and loneliness (Becker et al., 2021). Self-Determination Theory (SDT) on the other hand, founded on a wealth of research (Ryan et al., 2013) promotes autonomy (freedom to make our own decisions), relatedness or belonging (social significance and connection) and competence (efficacy and sense of control). Relatedness within the SDT model comes in the opposite spirit of disconnection and competition promoted by neoliberal ideology. The founders of SDT have worked with a moral philosopher to articulate the SDT vision and values

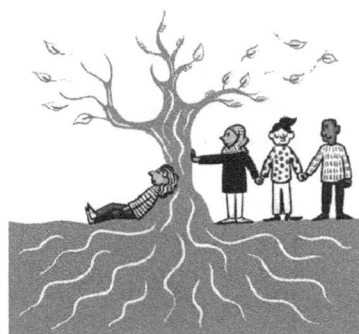
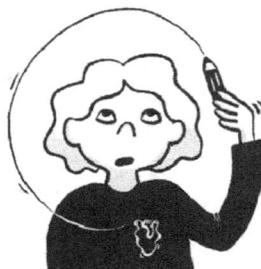

CREATING SPACES FOR PEOPLE TO SPEAK FROM THEIR HEART

SHARED MEANING MAKING

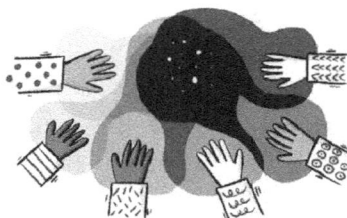

COMPASSION

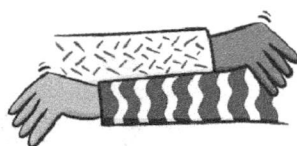

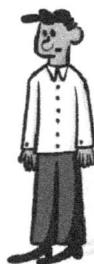

SHADOW WORK

Figure 12.4 Flourishing Model: Ecological, Making Connections, Shared Meaning Making, Compassion and Shadow Work (Younie 2023, 2024). (Illustrations © Camille Aubry, 2025, Used with Permission).

that align with human flourishing (Ryan et al., 2013). The authors evidence how intrinsic aspiration (valuing personal growth, relationship, community) which is in keeping with SDT and flourishing leads to higher wellbeing as compared to people holding extrinsic motivation (seeking rewards of success, money, fame – a more neoliberal framing) (Ryan et al., 2013). Further, employees who reported an intrinsic orientation evidenced greater satisfaction in their work, dedication and vitality and less emotional exhaustion (Ryan et al., 2013). Autonomy, Belonging and

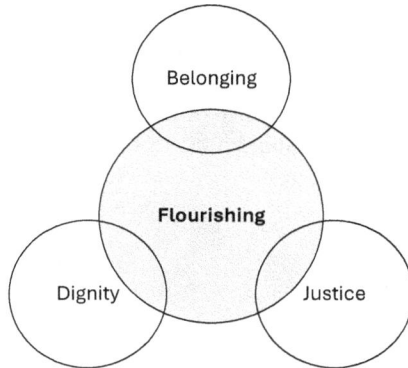

Figure 12.5 Belonging, Dignity, Justice and Flourishing (Younie, 2023).

Competence (as SDT is framed in GMCs Caring for Doctors Caring for Patients (West & Coia, 2019)) are however relatively thin on the ground in our modern day NHS in the UK, with similar pictures across the globe. Restoration of autonomy, for example, could involve giving doctors more flexibility in their schedule to allow for more individual styles of consultation, recognising the humanity and individuality of the patient and doctor (Hartzband & Groopman, 2020).

Another approach to flourishing we have been exploring locally, is an alternative model which emphasises the connection between Belonging, Dignity, Justice (BDJ) and flourishing: see Figure 12.5.

The BDJ model comes from Decolonise Design, a black led organisation (Davis, 2021) and takes a social justice stance. When belonging, dignity and justice are in harmony, we believe this to create what can be called a flourishing space. In a flourishing space, there is *Belonging* and space to question, share thoughts and reflect openly without fear of judgement. Listening to others, particularly those with different lived experiences, enables mutual enrichment and a broader, more inclusive understanding. Honouring the *Dignity* of ourselves or others relates to flourishing, where our imperfections are viewed through a generous appreciative lens, creating the space for personal and communal development. *Justice* provides the foundation for equal voice and equal value. Creating space to begin to see our own privileges or challenges alongside others may be uncomfortable but also necessary.

Conceptualisation of flourishing as a noun allows individual measurement of flourishing but risks missing injustice and social inequity as being barriers to flourishing. We align more with flourishing as a verb, i.e. to grow or develop within a congenial environment (Garland-Thomson, 2019), a way of travelling even through difficult challenges. In her research in the mid-west US, Willen et al found that some races and people in lower financial brackets were less likely to say they were flourishing (Willen et al., 2022). A critical approach such as that taken by Willen et al (Willen et al., 2022) aligns with our work and context at 'flourishing spaces.' By focussing on the spaces rather than on individuals, context and environment become relevant, allowing injustice in our systems to be more clearly seen. We are based in East London, the East side of cities in the UK traditionally being the poorer part where the fumes and pollution would blow, given the prevailing wind (Heblich et al., 2021). One of the core values of our institution, Queen Mary University of London (QMUL, 2019), is inclusion and widening participation. The flourishing spaces' values (below) have a critical edge, recognising that context, power and status have a huge influence on what individuals can achieve.

Flourishing spaces values

- Curiosity and epistemic humility: fostering a mindset open to the new, recognising that our own framing and ways of interpreting the world are socially constructed, rather than being absolute.
- Creative agency: moving from homo economicus, lonely and competitive, towards growing creative agency and voice, to challenge, question and bring creativity to our problem solving.
- Connection: catalysing relationship and community, recognising the value and need for bridge building.
- Compassion: recognising suffering and oppression, and actively working to relieve, enable and empower the suffering other as well as the suffering self.
- Co-creation: recognition of the value of shared agency, flattened hierarchy and systems thinking so that designing flourishing spaces will be enhanced by different parts of the system sharing their voices and perspectives.

The work is risky and requires inherent trust in our own humanity and that of others, but so too is any doctor-patient consultation, especially given the potential high vulnerability of our patients.

How do you know you have been in a flourishing space?

When we are in a space where we can risk being vulnerable, where the human dimension is valued with a recognition that we all struggle and fall short in different ways, and also where we can begin to find our unique voice, this is an emancipatory place where growth and flourishing might be enabled: see Figure 12.6. Here are three student quotes to illustrate these areas:

Vulnerability

The whole programme was very enjoyable, as I made friends who are understanding, kind and compassionate. With everyone, it felt safe to be vulnerable with each other, as everyone was willing to listen attentively and offer positive insight. Everyone was empathetic and offered unique perspectives during discussions, which was interesting to hear as everyone had different life experiences that influenced this (written reflection – flourishing through creative enquiry research, 2023).

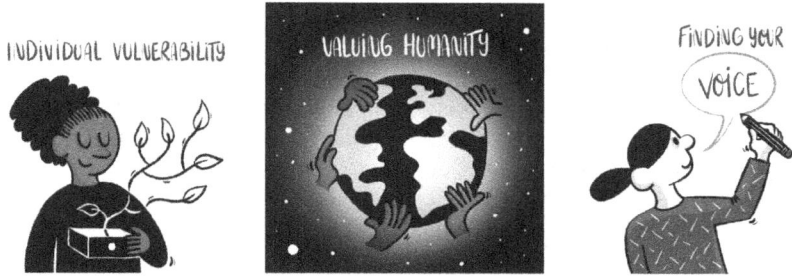

Figure 12.6 Vulnerability, Valuing Humanity, Voice (Aubry, 2025).

Value humanity

> …recognising the fact that many of us are broken actually and or have some weakness or something we've experienced that's been hurtful and we don't need to pretend that it's not there, we can, you know, we can live through that and be open about it when we want to be open about it. And that can actually be a way that we strengthen others or kind of open the possibility for them to share what they're going through and maybe be a support to them… (interview – flourishing through creative enquiry research, 2023).

Find voice

> …I think being creative can allow you to share your own thoughts with other people and it's … even for shy people, if they create something they don't … have to talk. They can let their creations speak for themselves. (interview – flourishing through creative enquiry research, 2023).

How might we create flourishing spaces in the neoliberal desert?

Creating a flourishing space requires a different kind of thinking to the thinking that has created our neoliberal spaces. I have created a 'toolkit' to support educator thinking about creating flourishing spaces for students, clinicians, patients, denoted with the acronym ASK… (Attend, Share stories and Shadow work and Kindle hope). The acronym also highlights the importance of asking. We may need to ask for space for our needs as humans and to have the courage to ask for help when we are struggling.

Attending to self and other

> Attention is the rarest and purest form of generosity
>
> (Simone Weil, 1976)

To attend to the self or the other means to be present, to listen, to witness. We can listen in order to learn from our patients or students; we can listen therapeutically, as well as to glean information. In the pressure of higher education or healthcare we may feel unseen and unheard whether clinician, educator, patient or student, and in the short space of the consultation, invaded with pop-ups on the computerised medical record, there is unlikely to be the 'mutual sighting' that DasGupta describes as necessary to the consultation (DasGupta, 2008). To counteract this, we may attend with a Beginner's Mind (Younie, 2017), a kind of hospitality where the other can dance their own dances (Nouwen, 1998), even if just for a brief moment. Fredrickson's research has demonstrated that the feeling of love even if very brief, enables a back-and-forth energy which blossoms virtually anytime two people connect in the presence of a shared positive emotion (Fredrickson, 2013). Unlike empathy alone, compassion triggers pleasure centres in the brain and there is evidence that it is linked with flourishing (Klimecki, 2012).

Attending may be supported by slowing down, using our senses and noticing. In the group setting, a facilitator may encourage relationships, psychological safety, valuing difference and diversity and encourage curiosity.

Sharing stories and shadow work

When we tell stories we move from two-dimensional to three-dimensional knowing, where we draw on our own inner seeing to create metaphors and symbols framing our view of the world. This can enhance understanding between two people with diverse and differing perspectives. Shadow work is possible when there is safety in the room and we are no longer pitched against each other in a competitive dance, but connected, communing.

In a group, I often invite people to choose a postcard that speaks to their lived experience and then to share it with two or three others in the room. This invites a time of quiet reflection and attending to self. As they begin to share their cards there is an attending to the other and the ways they frame the images on the card. Sharing stories often follows, in explanation of the images and ideas emerging. And at times depending on the quality of space and listening, stories of difficulties and challenges may emerge. Work is therefore needed in facilitation to give people permission to choose their own boundaries and how much they share both in the small group and back into the larger group.

Kindle hope

Whilst there is a literature on hope for our clinical practice with patients, little is written in terms of hope for healthcare professionals, struggling in the organisations and roles they find themselves in. Perhaps by reflecting on the starkest of situations, hope can be derived for the challenges we face in healthcare. In 'Man's Search for Meaning,' written by Viktor Frankl when he was interred in a concentration camp, Frankl describes how we can live with any 'how' if we can find a why (Frankl, 1992). By remaining committed to solidarity with his fellow prisoners, Frankl maintained a sense of meaning and purpose during his internment and went on to found a school of psychotherapy called 'logotherapy,' which attempts to help people rediscover meaning in their own lives.

Hope lies perhaps not in any individual's brilliance, but in the shared recognition of our challenges and mutual connection and collaboration in the face of what is messy and complex. Making space for building trust, encouraging friendship and collaboration, inviting creativity and participatory engagement, becoming a creative agent for change, and learning to welcome each small step as valuable for those lives it touches, may all increase our hope.

Limitations

The conceptualisation of flourishing is still in flux. There is a risk of 'flourishing' also serving a neoliberal agenda, whereby the most well-off flourish and find ways towards greater extrinsic reward. However, it is hard to imagine that we shouldn't aim to build relationships and community, to fight for justice, opposing oppression and to support and encourage others whenever we are able to.

What next

Creating flourishing spaces in healthcare is possible in any micro moment in any day. Each time we connect with a patient is a flourishing oasis from which both of us can drink, in what can otherwise feel like a parched terrain. Perhaps this recognition may help us to treasure that more dearly. As Scannell (2002) puts it:

> During "clinical hours" compressed into minutes by the exigencies of health care economics that drearily objectify us as "service providers", to articulate subjective experience— if even privately, if only momentarily—constitutes a radical act that defies this depersonalization.

Coaching, mentoring, supporting others also can provide sustaining nectar. More research is always needed; however, perhaps it is with creativity and innovation in practice that we need to extend the idea of flourishing spaces. Work is needed to transform cultures and systems, find language and create evidence for the human dimension of healthcare, and for human flourishing.

Conclusion

We are facing thirsty times in healthcare, both as patients and clinicians. In this chapter I have argued that neoliberalism has been a powerful force in shaping our reality and reducing space for us as human beings. We encourage resistance in the journey from homo economicus towards creative agent. Flourishing, meaning and purpose in our work may be costly, may incur the system's wrath, and yet may provide a regenerative approach towards wellbeing. My hope is to see many more flourishing oases opening up in the neoliberal desert, which sadly seems to be expanding alongside global warming. As one student put it:

> Flourishing really hits close to my heart, since I never thought of that mindset to view the world. I always felt pressured to be resilient – to not show my weakness but always put up a strong front.

(Hao, 2021)

References

Aubry, C. (2025). Illustrator at www.camilleaubry.com.

Asta, M., Milou, E. W. M. S., & Antonia, R. (2023). A national longitudinal cohort study of factors contributing to UK medical student's mental ill-health symptoms. *General Psychiatry, 36*(2), e101004. https://doi.org/10.1136/gpsych-2022-101004

Bansal, A., Greenley, S., Mitchell, C., Park, S., Shearn, K., & Reeve, J. (2022). Optimising planned medical education strategies to develop learners' person-centredness: A realist review. *Medical Education, 56*(5), 489–503. https://doi.org/https://doi.org/10.1111/medu.14707

Becker, J. C., Hartwich, L., & Haslam, S. A. (2021). Neoliberalism can reduce well-being by promoting a sense of social disconnection, competition, and loneliness. *British Journal of Social Psychology, 60*(3), 947–965. https://doi.org/https://doi.org/10.1111/bjso.12438

BMA. (2019). *Caring for the mental health of the medical workforce.* https://www.bma.org.uk/media/ckshvkzc/bma-mental-health-survey-report-september-2024.pdf

Brown, M. E. L., & Younie, L. (2022). How creative enquiry can help educators develop learners' person-centredness. *Medical Education, 56*(6), 599–601. https://doi.org/10.1111/medu.14794

Brown, W. (2015). *Undoing the demos: Neoliberalism's stealth revolution.* Princeton University Press.

Card, A. J. (2018). Physician burnout: Resilience training is only part of the solution. *Annals of Family Medicine, 16*(3), 267–270. https://doi.org/10.1370/afm.2223

Cribb, A., & Bignold, S. (1999). Towards the reflexive medical school: The hidden curriculum and medical education research. *Studies in Higher Education, 24,* 195–209. https://doi.org/10.1080/03075079912331379888   https://www.ingentaconnect.com/content/routledg/cshe/1999/00000024/00000002/art00005

DasGupta, S. (2008). Narrative humility. *Lancet, 371*(9617), 980–981. https://linkinghub.elsevier.com/retrieve/pii/S0140673608604407

Davis, A. M. (2021). *Diversity, equity and inclusion have failed. How about belonging, Dignity and justice instead?* https://www.weforum.org/stories/2021/02/diversity-equity-inclusion-have-failed-belonging-dignity-justice/

Dowrick, C., Heath, I., Hjörleifsson, S., Misselbrook, D., May, C., Reeve, J., Swinglehurst, D., & Toon, P. (2016). Recovering the self: A manifesto for primary care. *British Journal of General Practice, 66*(652), 582–583. https://doi.org/10.3399/bjgp16X687901

Dyrbye, L. N., Thomas, M. R., & Shanafelt, T. D. (2005). Medical student distress: Causes, consequences, and proposed solutions. *Mayo Clinic Proceedings, 80*(12), 1613–1622. https://doi.org/10.4065/80.12.1613

Fisher, J. A. (2007). Coming soon to a physician near you: Medical neoliberalism and pharmaceutical clinical trials. *Harvard Health Policy Review, 8*(1), 61–70.

Flickinger, T. E., Kon, R. H., Jacobsen, B., Schorling, J., May, N., Harrison, M., & Plews-Ogan, M. (2022). "Flourish in the clerkship year": A curriculum to promote wellbeing in medical students. *Medical Science Educator*, *32*(2), 315–320. https://doi.org/10.1007/s40670-022-01522-z

Frankl, V. E. (1992). *Man's search for meaning: An introduction to logotherapy*. Beacon Press.

Fredrickson, B. L. (2013). *Love 2.0: How our supreme emotion affects everything we feel, think, do, and become*. Hudson Street Press.

Fricker, M. (2007). *Epistemic injustice: Power & the ethics of knowing*. Oxford University Press.

Garland-Thomson, R. (2019). 15C1 welcoming the unexpected. In E. Parens & J. Johnston (Eds.), *Human flourishing in an age of gene editing* (pp. 15–28). Oxford University Press. https://doi.org/10.1093/oso/9780190940362.003.0002

Glaucomflecken. (2022, December 3). *How to fix burnout*. https://www.youtube.com/watch?v=MUVzRs3E5g4

Hao, Y. (2021). To flourish. *Journal of Holistic Healthcare*, *18*(2), 56.

Hartzband, P., & Groopman, J. (2020). Physician burnout, interrupted.*The New England Journal of Medicine*, *382*(26), 2485–2487. https://doi.org/10.1056/NEJMp2003149

Heath, I. (2018). Subjectivity of patients and doctors. In C. Dowrick (Ed.), *Person-centred primary care: Searching for the self* (pp. 77–98). Routledge.

Heblich, S., Trew, A., & Zylberberg, Y. (2021). East-side story: Historical pollution and persistent neighborhood sorting. *Journal of Political Economy*, *129*(5), 1508–1552. https://doi.org/10.1086/713101

Huta, V. (2015). The complementary roles of eudaimonia and hedonia and how they can be pursued in practice. In S. Joseph (Ed.), *Positive psychology in practice : Promoting human flourishing in work, health, education, and everyday life* (pp. 159–182). John Wiley & Sons, Inc.

Ichioka, S., & Pawlyn, M. (2021). *Flourish: Design paradigms for our planetary emergency*. Triarchy Press.

Illing, J. (2007). *Thinking about research: Frameworks, ethics and scholarship*. Newcastle University.

Jung, C. G. (2014). *The archetypes and the collective unconscious*. Routledge.

Keyes, C. L. (2002). The mental health continuum: From languishing to flourishing in life. *Journal of Health and Social Behavior*, *43*(2), 207–222. https://www.ncbi.nlm.nih.gov/pubmed/12096700

Klein, N. (2007). *The shock doctrine: The rise of disaster capitalism*. Knopf Canada.

Klimecki, O. (2012). *Empathy and compassion in society*. https://www.youtube.com/watch?v=GxH-Oiqz-14

Levin, J. (2021). Human flourishing: A new concept for preventive medicine. *American Journal of Preventative Medicine*, *61*(5), 761–764.

Mate, G. (2019). *How culture makes us feel lost - Dr. Gabor Maté on finding your true self again*. Retrieved 03/12/2024 from https://www.youtube.com/watch?v=TIjvXtZRerY

Mavelli, L. (2019). Resilience beyond neoliberalism? Mystique of complexity, financial crises, and the reproduction of neoliberal life. *Resilience*, *7*(3), 224–239. https://doi.org/10.1080/21693293.2019.1605661

Metcalf, S. (2017). Neoliberalism: The idea that swallowed the world. *The Guardian*. https://www.theguardian.com/news/2017/aug/18/neoliberalism-the-idea-that-changed-the-world

Monbiot, G. (2016). Neoliberalism – the ideology at the root of all our problems. *The Guardian*. https://www.theguardian.com/books/2016/apr/15/neoliberalism-ideology-problem-george-monbiot

Nouwen, H. J. M. (1998). *Reaching out* (3rd ed.). Fount Paperbacks.

Panagioti, M., Geraghty, K., Johnson, J., Zhou, A., Panagopoulou, E., Chew-Graham, C., Peters, D., Hodkinson, A., Riley, R., & Esmail, A. (2018). Association between physician burnout and patient safety, professionalism, and patient satisfaction: A systematic review and meta-analysis. *JAMA Internal Medicine, 178*(10), 1317–1330. https://doi.org/10.1001/jamainternmed.2018.3713

QMUL. (2019). Strategy 2030: *Queen Mary 2030: The most inclusive university of its kind, anywhere*. Queen Mary University of London.

Ryan, R. M., Current, R. R., & Deci, E. L. (2013). What humans need: Flourishing in Aristotelian philosophy and self-determination theory. In A. S. Waterman (Ed.), *The best within us: Positive psychology perspectives on eudaimonia* (pp. 57–75). American Psychological Association. https://doi.org/10.1037/14092-004

Scannell, K. (2002). Writing for our lives: Physician narratives and medical practice. *Annals of Internal Medicine, 137*(9), 779–781. PM:12416971 (NOT IN FILE)

Seligman, M. (2011). *Flourish: A visionary new understanding of happiness and well-being*. Free Press.

Shanafelt, T. D., Balch, C. M., Bechamps, G., Russell, T., Dyrbye, L., Satele, D., Collicott, P., Novotny, P. J., Sloan, J., & Freischlag, J. (2010). Burnout and medical errors among American surgeons. *Annals of Surgery, 251*(6), 995–1000. https://doi.org/10.1097/SLA.0b013e3181bfdab3

Sinskey, J. L., Margolis, R. D., & Vinson, A. E. (2022). The wicked problem of physician well-being. *Anesthesiology Clinics, 40*(2), 213–223. https://doi.org/10.1016/j.anclin.2022.01.001

Slavin, S. J., Hatchett, L., Chibnall, J. T., Schindler, D., & Fendell, G. (2011). Helping medical students and residents flourish: A path to transform medical education. *Academic Medicine, 86*(11), e15. https://doi.org/10.1097/ACM.0b013e3182316558

Spiro, H. (2004). The accurate eye, the truthful ear. *The Yale Journal for Humanities in Medicine*.

Taylor, R. A. (2019). Contemporary issues: Resilience training alone is an incomplete intervention. *Nurse Education Today, 78*, 10–13. https://doi.org/https://doi.org/10.1016/j.nedt.2019.03.014

Teodorczuk, A., Thomson, R., Chan, K., & Rogers, G. D. (2017). When I say … resilience. *Medical Education, 51*(12), 1206–1208. https://doi.org/10.1111/medu.13368

Tilburt, J., & Geller, G. (2007). Viewpoint: The Importance of worldviews for medical education. *Academic Medicine, 82*(8), 819–822. https://doi.org/10.1097/ACM.0b013e3180d098cc

Van der Kolk, B. (2014). *The body keeps the score. Mind, brain and body in the transformation of trauma*. Viking Penguin.

VanderWeele, T. J. (2017). On the promotion of human flourishing. *Proceedings of the National Academy of Sciences of the United States of America, 114*(31), 8148–8156. https://doi.org/10.1073/pnas.1702996114

Weil, S. (1976). *Simone Weil: A life* (S. Pétrement, Ed.; R. Rosenthal, Trans., p. 105). Pantheon Books.

West, C. P., Dyrbye, L. N., Sinsky, C., Trockel, M., Tutty, M., Nedelec, L., Carlasare, L. E., & Shanafelt, T. D. (2020). Resilience and burnout among physicians and the general US working population. *JAMA Network Open, 3*(7), e209385. https://doi.org/10.1001/jamanetworkopen.2020.9385

West, M., & Coia, D. (2019). *Caring for doctors, caring for patients: How to transform UK healthcare environments to support doctors and medical students to care for patients*. General Medical Council.

Whitaker, R. C., Payne, G. B., O'Neill, M. A., Brennan, M. M., Herman, A. N., Dearth-Wesley, T., & Weil, H. F. C. (2024). Trauma-informed undergraduate medical education: A pathway to flourishing with adversity by enhancing psychological safety. *Perspectives on Medical Education, 13*(1), 324–331. https://doi.org/10.5334/pme.1173

Willen, S. S., Williamson, A. F., Walsh, C. C., Hyman, M., & Tootle, W. (2022). Rethinking flourishing: Critical insights and qualitative perspectives from the U.S. Midwest. *SSM - Mental Health, 2*, 100057. https://doi.org/10.1016/j.ssmmh.2021.100057

Younie, L. (2014). Arts-based inquiry and a clinician educator's journey of discovery. In C. L. McLean (Ed.), *Creative arts in humane medicine* (pp. 163–180). Brush Education Inc.

Younie, L. (2016). Vulnerable leadership. *London Journal of Primary Care, 8*(3), 37–38. https://doi.org/10.1080/17571472.2016.1163939

Younie, L. (2017). Beginner's mind. *London Journal of Primary Care, 9*(6), 83–85. https://doi.org/10.1080/17571472.2017.1370768

Younie, L. (2019). Vulnerability, resilience and the arts. In J. Patterson & F. Kinchington (Eds.), *Body talk: Whose language?* (pp. 64–77). Cambridge Scholars.

Younie, L. (2020). When I say flourishing in medical education… *Journal of Holistic Healthcare, 17*(3), 44–46.

Younie, L. (2021a). Flourishing through creative enquiry: Humanising the medical experience. *Journal of Holistic Healthcare, 18*(1), 3–5.

Younie, L. (2021b). Humanising medical education. *Journal of Holistic Healthcare, 18*(3), 37–39.

Younie, L. (2021c). What does creative enquiry have to contribute to flourishing in medical education? In E. Murray & J. Brown (Eds.), *The mental health and wellbeing of healthcare practitioners: Research and practice* (pp. 14–27). Wiley-Blackwell.

Younie, L. (2023). *Flourishing.* www.creativeenquiry.co.uk

Younie, L. (2024). How might we cultivate flourishing spaces? *Journal of Holistic Healthcare, 21*(1), 14–16.

13 Quality rebellion

Hermeneutics beyond the clinical encounter

Jane Myat and Jane Riddiford

Jane Myat has been a GP at the same practice in north London for 27 years. Drawing on her own experiences, knowing that there is more to health than can be delivered in the confines of the consulting room, Jane worked alongside her patients and members of the local community to create a garden in the middle of her group practice. This became known as The Listening Space. Working in and with that space opened up practical possibilities to explore questions: what it is to be well, how we might heal ourselves, each other and the natural world. It also led to meeting others travelling with the same enquiries in the local area.

Jane Riddiford has a wealth of experience in creating the conditions for good community. Her work has involved growing an urban forest in Auckland, working with story, whether that be in street theatre or in circles in many different places. Jane co-founded the charity, Global Generation in London, bringing environmental education to young people, their families and the local community. Jane has returned to her native New Zealand and co-founded Ruamāhanga Farm Foundation, a community-oriented wetland and riparian forest restoration project.

Introduction

The words rebel, revolution and revolt share a common Latin ancestry – rebellare, revolutio, revolvere – each carrying the essence of breaking boundaries. These words evoke disruption, resistance and expression – energies turned towards transformation, often in defiance of authority or oppression. And radical is derived from *radicalis*: from the roots, the ground, vital to life, searching.

In 'Why We Revolt,' Victor Montori, physician and founder of The Patient Revolution, illuminates how the industrialisation of healthcare has warped its core mission (Montori, 2020). He argues that healthcare has ceased to care, becoming a machine more concerned with efficiency than humanity. His call is simple: we must transform healthcare from an industrial activity to a deeply human one that provides careful and kind care for all. *'The difference between what is and what should be,'* he writes, *'provides voltage to a revolution.'*

As the system has eroded, so too has its language. 'Quality' has been reduced to a business metric, locked into rigid, hollowed-out terms: access, efficiency, value, clinical outcomes, safety, patient satisfaction. This is lifeless, Orwellian

DOI: 10.4324/9781003517665-13

doublespeak at odds with any true sense of excellence. And consider the word 'healthcare' itself. As we pull things apart, separate and divide, where has the health gone and where is the care? Can we reunite, restore and revive, making healthcare meaningfully whole again?

In the writing that follows, we invite you to explore health as a living, breathing relationship, rooted in our cells and extending outwards into our bodies, communities, and the ecosystems that sustain us. To care is to pay attention, to see, to listen, to feel. Care becomes compassion when we connect with the joy and suffering of others because we realise: there is no 'other.' We are all interconnected.

The concept of 'quality rebels' was first introduced by Dutch management scholar Jules Goddard in the early 2000s. He described these individuals as those who challenge the status quo, not for the sake of opposition but to drive meaningful improvements. In healthcare, quality rebellion, championed by thinkers like Wallenburg et al. (2019), questions established norms, pushes boundaries and advocates for change, with the ultimate goal of improving care. This rebellion is the lifeblood of innovation and creativity, necessary for any system seeking to remain flexible, energised and vital.

Just as rewilding movements restore balance to ecosystems, quality rebellion in healthcare seeks to challenge rigid norms and outdated processes. It envisions health as a vast system that extends beyond individuals to include the land, water, and communities that are essential to life itself. Quality rebellion may address root causes: polluted rivers, depleted soils, broken social structures. As rivers regain their natural flow through re-wiggling (Saunders, 2023), healthcare too can find new vitality-unlocking creativity, embracing flexibility and healing at its core. It's a path towards regenerative health, not just for individuals, but for the planet too. This path can provide new perspectives and new meanings for those who take it.

An invitation

In the spirit of rebellion, this chapter may take on a less familiar form than its predecessors. We begin it together, speaking as one voice, before inviting you to follow the tributaries of our individual stories. In the end, we will come back together to reflect on what we've learned from our separate yet intertwined paths.

We encourage you to slow down, to embrace the turning points and vistas that arise on your own journey. In a world that moves too quickly, it's easy to forget that the most meaningful part of any journey isn't the destination, but the experiences along the way. We have found that time spent in the realm of story, as well as time spent in the depths of nature can help the business of making meaning and finding ways for mending and repair, especially in a world that often feels chaotic and broken.

> After nourishment, shelter and companionship, stories are what we need most in the world
>
> (Phillip Pullman, date unknown)

Setting out: our story

We met accidentally in one of Global Generation's Skip Gardens and soon bonded through our respective interest in the connections between habitat, natural spaces and health. We were both interested in edgelands and borders: the liminal spaces where change and transformation occur. We found common ground, perhaps most importantly a 'wayfinding' practice. This approach is inspired by the early Pacific explorers, the wayfinders, who without instruments to measure, found their way forward through relying on multiple forms of intelligence. As leadership scholar Chellie Spiller and her co-authors describe in the book Wayfinding Leadership (2015), *'this kind of navigation requires us to set sail beyond the scope of our imaginations.'*

Neither of us are researchers in the conventional sense; we are very much practitioners with a common affinity to action research approaches:

> Action research seeks to bring together action and reflection, theory and practice, in participation with others in the pursuit of practical solutions to issues of pressing concern to people and more generally the flourishing of persons and their communities.
>
> (Reason & Bradbury, 2001)

This actively enquiring path underpinned how we navigated our multi-layered relationship as patient and doctor, neighbours, friends and participants in community projects.

In 2020, the COVID-19 pandemic crept into London, with all of its strangeness and suffering, along with unexpected pockets of reprieve. As the air cleared and the sound of the birdsong grew, a space opened up for us to collaborate more formally than we had before, driven by a wish to address the rising sense of pressure and uncertainty in ourselves and those we were involved with. One of our responses was to create a series of Story Walks through the green spaces of Camden. In time we realised that we had been walking along the path of the buried River Fleet, which was once called the Holy River of Wells.

These tiny journeys of sanctuary nurtured our shared belief in the healing power of story. Our weekly walks extended over two years. As we moved between green and blue spaces in the city, we shared tales, writing, poetry, art and music. The pandemic had provided a pause, a place ripe with possibility, the chance to find our way into more hopeful stories. We travelled with our questions: What is the healing power of a river? How might we regenerate at this time of transition? How might we let go of what is ending and allow ourselves to open to new beginnings? Often our walks started in the Listening Space Garden in Kentish Town and finished in the Story Garden in King's Cross. As we walked, talked and moved in silence we shifted to a slower gear and got to know each other and the world around us in new ways. Through paying attention to the big and the small, be it a childhood memory or an ailing tree, we became more keenly aware of the healing power of the physical and the metaphorical landscape we all inhabit.

Since that time, thresholds, change and transformation have come in other forms too. We now live on opposite sides of the globe, Jane having returned to her native Aotearoa, New Zealand. Despite the thousands of miles between us, we remain in regular dialogue. Over time in our imaginations and our practice in different parts of the world, the footprints left by the Story Walks morphed into the narrative notion of a River of Hope, the name we now give to an annual collaboration of community groups in a spirit of health, creativity and celebration.

Over the last few years of our partnership, writing and exchanging our newly minted words has been a way of making meaning. In writing this chapter, we hoped we would surprise ourselves and discover something new, rather than recycling what we already knew. As a way of starting, we invited each other to write about what our hands had been doing in the last few days.

Jane M – These hands

I waved my brown and now wrinkly hands in front of me as I announced:

These hands have baked cakes for you to enjoy today.

This was how I introduced myself to a small delegation of health professionals who were part of an MBA program at the Rotman Business School in Canada. They were visiting our Listening Space garden for a third year as part of a field trip, exploring aspects of UK health systems. I'm not sure how we are presented on their program. Something of an alternative, grassroots, social prescribing project in action perhaps. I passed the baton and the circle of smiling faces readily joined in:

These hands have held many dying hands/ delivered lots of babies into the world/ love to tickle piano keys/ tap away for far too long on my keyboard/ have held my children's hands/ love to weave/ to sew/to grow. These hands have the power to lower people's blood pressure

In this way, we allowed the human dimension gently in and found out more about the people gathered than we might have, had we asked them to introduce themselves in a more customary fashion. We already knew we were amongst people working variously as clinicians, managers or in other roles in our modern healthcare industry. The question invited them to step outside our 'flat-pack' world into one of vibrancy, texture and colour.

The Rotman visit had been looming in my diary as another bittersweet stepping stone on the journey I was making towards leaving the practice I had been working in for the last 27 years: a complex decision which came fast and slow and full of mixed emotions. I was going through a giant breakup making me question my identity, what I was doing in making this change, unsure about all that had gone before and might come next. And at the risk of sounding dramatic, I felt a little like I was dying. Something was dissolving inside of me. This was chrysalid time, messy but with potential. It was a curious feeling. An emptying of neglected cupboards. Disturbance, disruption, dust, debris, detritus, grief. And unspeakable dread. A threshold. A place where the undergirding current was shifting and I was struggling to keep afloat. I experienced a reversal of roles. My patients now brought me care, thanks, stories and support. It is usually my place to be the ballast, steadying others whilst things fall apart.

In sage and wise medicine, GPs are guardians: not just keepers of stories but also of gates, accompanying people back and forth across the borderlands separating dis-ease and disease. Conduits, edge-dwellers, channels and pores. We stitch together stories, blending the mythic and scientific. We are creatively frugal using time, trust and relationship as people bring us their material. Kaleidoscopes of colours, textures of all types from the sturdy, hard-wearing, here-to-stay fabrics to the ephemeral, fragile whispering fragments still searching for a place to land. My life has been spent patiently mending and repairing. I weave, making connections, putting pieces together. Regularly shifting perspective, moving in and out, looking for patterns, finding a place for the different pieces. And over time, a patchworked cloth grows in me telling the tales of humanity and hardship, of beauty and brokenness: a cloak of protection full of wisdom, to be offered as shelter and comfort for those who come visiting next.

I turn this cloth over in my mind and think of all the patients I've been privileged to see and hear over all these years. When they heard I was leaving, many came to see me to reminisce about the times we've shared. They knew I carry their stories. We had encountered thresholds together, when the narrative flow of life took a turn, or the way forward was not clear. We had travelled through beginnings and endings, pregnancies and births, dying and deaths as well as loss in its many forms. We had been at the edge, when life no longer looked predictable. But we all secretly know that predictability is an illusion anyway: the dream net we cast to create a sense of safety that allows us to carry on, to keep the awe out.

I had been hearing too in my leaving what had mattered in those clinical encounters.

Thank you for all your care/ your kindness/ for making me feel safe/ for looking me in the eyes and really seeing me/ for listening/ for being there/ for your accompaniment

Interestingly I hadn't had expressions of gratitude for getting someone's blood pressure or cholesterol below target or prescribing the right medicine, though of course, that is all part of the medical role. But what matters goes far beyond that: treasuring the whole person, not just measuring what we can of their physical body. The welcome, hospitality and attention needed to really 'see' someone close-up. This is the sanctuary space of care. The love that is necessary for true healing work.

Whilst contemplating how to make meaning of my own life in medicine, I stood in front of the Rotman group and looked again at my hands. I told them the story of how my hands had linked with many other hands in starting our Listening Space garden. I told them this was 'woumbed' from 'lovage': a play on words to hold something of the creation that occurs when the seeming opposites of love and rage meet. The garden was birthed from my wounding by the harshness of the medical world and driven by a heady mixture of love for my people and rage at the machine. I was full of grief at the time, following a string of bereavements, my world turned upside down. I could no longer remain within the lines drawn by The System: meet-measure-move on. Faster and faster. Suffocated by the infestation of rapidly multiplying tiny-tick-boxes, the blur and the speed were making me and my patients sick. It felt deliciously rebellious to escape the confines of the industrialised consulting room, away from conveyor-belt medicine and into the open air. To outside observers I am sure that creating the garden looked chaotic. But it was a fertile tumbling, which led to a roar of flowers echoing around the courtyard walls and plunging through this patch of uncherished land at the centre of our urban practice. We pushed ourselves up through cracks in the concrete, dreaming and playing our way to new possibilities. This was the magic we needed to heal our alienation and despair, the re-enchantment that allowed healing. A connection with the pattern of creation – growing roots, re-membering, connecting, forming networks, appreciating our diversity.

Replacing boundaries with 'near-carefulness'

Creating the Listening Space was a time of rapid change and although turbulent, there was an energy in the rebellion that propelled me forwards and opened the way to more experimentation. My relationships with my patients changed, power shifted and we worked more collaboratively together. We grew in confidence so that it became safe to fail but always good to try new things and different ways of working, as long as we were grounded by our values and able to have open and honest dialogue with each other. Jo Lynch, a former patient at the practice and now one of our generous social prescribers, initiated a supportive crafting circle that still meets weekly after several years. Many, including reception staff look forward to 'Crafternoons' with their transformational effect on our waiting room and relationships.

Over the years since we began, we have held lots of celebratory events. It makes me wonder if we should be thought of as quality 'revels,' not rebels. Through cooking, singing and dancing together, we have grown our relational network and discovered our shared humanity. A common concern is that this activity oversteps boundaries that should exist between clinician and patient. Iona Heath (2024) in her book, 'John Berger,' reflects on the Icelandic word *nær-gœtni:* 'apparently it means near-carefulness – the care that needs to be taken when one comes near to another.' And it is precisely this more porous, responsive near-carefulness that I realised we need to cultivate rather than solely relying on the protection of rigid professional distance to avoid potential boundary transgressions. 'Near-carefulness' allows us to more respectfully see, hear and delight in the other. It was this approach that allowed me to invite my distressed, self-harming patient to repurpose the negative energy of her cutting into the positive act of chopping and helping Jo to prepare the staff's weekly lunch one day. This turned out to be a rapid, generative and transformational intervention as an alternative to sending her to the crisis house again.

The patient in question grew in confidence and subsequently completed a culinary qualification. I told the Rotman group that we specialise in 'possibilitation.'

Reminded by Jane of Sand Talk, I re-read Tyson Yunkaporta's (2019) invitational book which explores how indigenous thinking can save the world.

> I yarn about what I call rigak lokath- the brackish water formed in the wet season when the fresh water floods down the rivers into the saltwater along the coast ... a phenomenon of dynamic interaction occurring when opposite forces meet in an act of new creation. It is a principle that guides the interactions of different groups and interests in society, a reflection of the natural processes of self-organising systems. Changes and transformations occur this way. Dynamic systems of culture, events and languages evolve over time through this interaction

How do we achieve balance, marry constancy and change? Silent walks with Jane on Hampstead Heath and winter swimming developed into our Story Walks during which our imaginations grew wings. We could feel the buried river Fleet coming back to the surface of the land. All that we'd forgotten, we felt arising too. There were tears of grief and of praise. As the River of Hope rose, it became the theme for our community party both across the borough of Camden and twinned now with Jane's wetland and riparian forest restoration project in Aotearoa, New Zealand. Global Generation explored the story further through their Voices of the Water project.

In thinking about writing our chapter in this book about meaning making, themes emerged about the liminal: spaces of transition and transformation. How do we find our way, make sense when things don't make sense? I think this is the brackish meeting place that Yunkaporta describes. A place where things collide: the whirlpools created when opposing flows meet, creating flux and transformation; the cosmic dance that moves forwards and back from chaos and disorder into pattern and rhythm. I was reminded of the experiment where metronomes are set off at random times, but quickly come into synchrony: the spell of the relational, the same magic that is harnessed in traditional healing. I contemplated the central importance of story, belief, ritual and ceremony to hold us. I read about wounded healers meeting wounded storytellers (Frank, 1995) at a time when I was encountering transition and transformation of my own.

David Abram in his essay 'The Ecology of Magic' (Abram, 1995) explores the connection between folk-medicine and magic:

> The traditional magician, I came to discern, commonly acts as an intermediary between the human collective and the larger ecological field, ensuring that there is an appropriate flow of nourishment, not just from the landscape to the human inhabitants but from the human community back to the local Earth.

I wonder when we lost our perspective, our link with the pattern of the universe, our place in the order of things, our humility, healthy doubt and respect for mystery? As these questions surfaced again in me, I sensed a now familiar tension arising, filling me up. Experience told me another story was about to be told in my own life. Much like the release of the waters from a previously culverted river. Katherine May (2023), in *Enchantment: reawakening wonder in an anxious age*, writes:

> There has been a yearning in me that I'm only just beginning to understand, a craving for transcendent experience, for depth, for meaning-making. It's not just that the world needs to change - I need to change, too. I need to soften, to let go of the tight empirical boundaries, to find a greater fluidity in my being.

One of the delegates from the Rotman group asked me about how we might 'scale our innovation.' It was not the first time I had been asked this. It's an itchy and uncomfortable question. I didn't set out to create 'a thing.' What came had its own life: something embodied, powerful. I let go and it took me over. It was intuitive. My heart and my hands knew what they wanted to do and where they wanted to go. My 'head' and the articulation came later. I don't like the word 'scaling,' it carries connotations of the corporate machine: capturing, dissecting, reducing to extract material towards a product. Often, the end result is a lifeless imitation of something once vital. So instead of scaling and building lego-like structures, can we allow a more organic growth as Jeynine Benyus' proposes in her book, Biomimicry (Benyus, 1997)? Here she asks us to contemplate whether we might find solutions to human challenges by learning to imitate nature's 3.8 billion years of research and development. Might we then be on a safari towards optimal form, function, process, system or strategy?

I reframe the question of scaling. How might we grow, flourish and ignite vitality in our projects and lives, especially when navigating a world filled with uncertainty? This question has been with me for a long time, and I've been quietly holding one of the answers, though unsure if I should share it. It wriggled in my pocket, whispering insistently, urging me to bring it out. I hesitated – would it sound strange? Would anyone understand? But the squirming wouldn't stop. I pulled out a pack of playing cards and began to tell their story.

These may seem like ordinary playing cards, but they are cards with a difference. My husband, Simon, a child and adolescent psychiatrist, and I designed this pack together. Hidden within their simplicity is wisdom foraged from years lived in medicine and the world of ideas. They are here to challenge a materialistic culture that prizes the external over the internal. These cards invite you to reflect, to soften your thoughts in times of uncertainty – because to change the world, we must first change how we think. Inspired by manomaya, a concept from Indian philosophy, these cards, which we call *The CARDS* (Myat et al., 2024), are both playful and profound – 'tools for navigating what it means to be human.'

The CARDS emerged during a time of immense pressure for our family, when we were thrown into a storm of uncertainty and faced our own mortality. In that crucible, the impulse to create something meaningful took root. These cards are our offering, our way of saying, *we were here*. They are the result of a lifetime of listening, of distilling experiences as wounded healers who have been entrusted with the stories of others. In a world that has lost many of its shared rituals and ceremonies,

The CARDS are an invitation to gather around a table, to reconnect with each other and with ourselves. They are tools for sparking 'conversations inviting change' (Launer, 2018), supporting us in our shared exploration of more integrated ways of being.

We used an ordinary pack of playing cards as the frame to organise some of the elements needed for an inner journey. With the help of the talented local artist Chrissie Nicholls, we embedded tracks and clues within her beautiful illustrations. Together, we condensed our story into 52 cards: red and black for polarities such as day and night; four suits for the seasons; 365, their sum total representing the passing of days. *The CARDS* are designed to spark a different kind of conversation, to invite active participation, and perhaps take us into uncharted waters, to places of discovery.

I described how I had been sharing *The CARDS* with some of my patients, reminding them that everything they need is already within. But when they lose their way, *The CARDS* are there to whisper a path back home. They can act as a transitional object, bridging the space between us and touching something deeper, something universal. As I gift packs to departing Rotman delegates, I slip the King of Hearts: The Threshold Card, from my own pack into my pocket after sending a photograph of it to Jane. Sharing this story has allowed me to reflect, to gaze both backwards and forwards, and to wonder what my hands will create next.

Jane R – picking up the thread

I look at my phone, taking in a photograph of what looks like a woven platter held by different hands. The pattern of the weaving reminds me of the spiralled lines and spaces that sit at the heart of a tree; marks that are old and still shaping. It is the image of the threshold card that Jane has sent me.

In a few days' time, we will be hosting a group of students for a learning and volunteering day. They are from a conservation course run by Pūkaha, a local bird sanctuary. Whilst I have run many similar education days at our gardens in London, this is my first time doing something like that here at Ruamāhanga Farm. I feel all the anxiety that goes with any threshold moment. My worries are heightened by the fact that my husband Rod's health has not been great. Pūkaha is on land traditionally owned by Rangatāne o Wairarapa, one of the two local tribes in our valley.

In recent years, with the resurgence in Te ao Maori (a Maori world view), customary protocols designed to bring people together with a sense of respect and meaning have become more widely practised. A few months ago, I participated in an overnight environmental education hui; a meeting to discuss issues of community concern at Pūkaha. The event was threaded through with time-honoured rituals, some of which resonated with the action research informed ways of meaning making we applied in Global Generation's gardens in London and now here at Ruamāhabga Farm. Like the spiralled patterns in a tree, they are rituals that are old and still shaping. At the hui and other similar events, before hearing about anybody's role in their various organisations, we heard about the mountain, the river and the sea, that the ancestors of the people in the group came from including the sea faring vessel the ancestors travelled to Aotearoa on, for all of us here are immigrants. Little more than 1000 years ago, there were only birds on these islands. The proceedings were gentle and inclusive, encouraging those of us not so embedded in the Māori world to take part. The invitation encouraged us to honour the land and the waters that have shaped us and was a powerful way of slowing down and building trust.

In the days preceding the Pūkaha students' visit to Ruamāhanga Farm, my planning spanned different spheres. I thought about how to prepare both the earth and the atmosphere between us. Rod and I walked the land and identified the places the students would clear in preparation for children from a local primary school to plant trees and grasses the following week. We thought about the order of the day and how to orchestrate spaces for the stories we hoped the students would share. Before hearing about the places our guests were from, I decided to invite them to share a karakia, a chanted prayer (Marsden, 2003).

I became more keenly aware of introducing steps to bring the energy up and down throughout the day. I felt grateful for the writing and reflecting Jane and I had been doing and even appreciative of Rod's low energy situation. It meant that I had gone more carefully and considerately than I might otherwise have done. My thoughts turned to food as a way of grounding the group and making them feel welcome. As I imagined the lunch and the afternoon tea, I felt in step with Jane and all the meals and afternoon teas I had enjoyed with her in The Listening Space garden. For our day with the students, we would have soup, bread and a cake to end the day. Before the afternoon activity of envisaging how to begin restoring a fragile wetland, we would make time for our guests to sit quietly beside the flowing waters of the Rumāhanga River. Time for a 'glistening tears' river story; one that grew from a chief's journey through the shapes and time-worn markings of our valley. Time to slow down and listen to what the river might have to say. In that way, on that day, we would bring to life the River of Hope.

Jane M – sedimenting

My hands were still, I needed to sit, to quieten and slow at this point of change in my life, at the end of this chapter, not quite knowing what would come next, with a concern for what our lives and our children's lives might hold. I was reminded of the words of Bayo Akomolafe 'The times are urgent: let us slow down' *(Akomolafe)*.

I reached for the card I put in my pocket the day before. The 'Threshold Card' was inspired by Dougald Hine's book, At Work in the Ruins (Hine, 2023), to offer support when you might otherwise feel lost. There are questions here and an image of two sets of hands holding/sharing/handing over a basket.

Before crossing the threshold of this journey, pause. What will I take with me? What will I leave behind? What might I have forgotten?

As I left the practice, I gave thanks for all the stories I would take with me along with the invisible threads of connections that continue to bind me to my community.

I thought of the reciprocity of giving and receiving, like the hands holding this basket. A reminder too that although transition and change can be frightening, we are not alone. We can be each other's wind resistance. I had been clearing my office, creating dust, sorting, surfacing and sedimenting. I wondered what I might have forgotten? I smiled. I was lightening my load for this next part of my journey. To leave space in the basket, an empty pocket: room to breathe.

Reflections: transitions, transformations, endings and beginnings

We live in a time of great noise and unprecedented peril, when the threads that connect us feel fragile. The world is growing hotter: inflammatory conditions overtaking our bodies, conflicts fracturing our communities and rising global temperatures threatening all life on earth. It is all too easy to succumb to fear and paralysis in the face of such crises. Central to our practice is the shared conviction that if we can find ways to come together, we can offer each other the shelter and sanctuary we need to settle and quieten.

Macy and Brown (2014) calls this *The Great Turning* a moment where we can shift the narrative from extraction and separation to one of healing and regeneration. Can we awaken from the story of endless growth and destruction? Can we find our way back to the earth, to each other, and to the wisdom of interconnection?

At these threshold moments, it can be helpful to look both backwards and forwards, whilst grounding ourselves in the radical gift of the present. For most of human history, we have balanced two essential ways of knowing: *mythos* and *logos*. Through the stories we told each other and within our communities we learned more about how *mythos* is the voice of the unconscious, a voice that speaks to the timeless dimensions of who we are. These stories helped us make meaning from chaos, guiding us through grief and sorrow. In this process of making room for all ways of knowing we also welcomed *logos*, the rational mind which holds the power to drive us to act, to control, to order the world around us. However in a world *dominated* by *logos*, we have a pressing need to reclaim story and meaning making, to restore balance.

What else did we learn from our journey? What practices helped us nurture the conditions for good health of both land and people? Though we now work in different physical landscapes and communities, we are still shaped by the same metaphorical terrain. This shared landscape continues to guide us, offering sustenance and direction through the rhythms of nature and the old stories, tales shaped both by the land itself and by the people who lived in deep harmony with it.

David Abram (1997) reminds us:

> There was a time when human beings were much more intimately involved in the landscape, where our very language mimicked and was developed from the movement of the earth itself.

The stories we have shared are not just our own. They are part of a broader tide of renewal. Quality rebellion is not about heroics but about leaning into the wind, feeling the pressure and linking arms with others who sense the same currents.

It means holding fear in the one hand and courage in the other, daring to challenge the entrenched ways we think about health, community and care.

When the systems around us falter, no longer serving the whole, we turn to the weather of change. We stand resilient in the storm, doing what we can to provide shelter and steadfastness during turbulent times. Quality rebellion is not merely disruption; it is attunement to suffering, driven by an inner sense of interconnection and responsibility. It is a refusal to turn away from pain, accompanied by the resolve to respond with care.

Rebels of quality are not just disruptors but creators, navigating the rivers of transformation with the intention to mend and renew. Their actions are rooted in a deep care for people and planet, recognising that the wellbeing of both is intertwined. In this way, rebellion becomes a generative act. It is a conscious commitment to fostering flourishing and regeneration, to nurturing life in all its intricate and fragile beauty.

We learned by doing, by trying and reflecting. And we were prepared to unlearn as much as we learned. This is at the heart of the way we practise *action research*. It has been a guiding and evolving methodology that calls us to engage directly with the messy realities of the world, rather than working from a place of fixed knowledge or certainty. In terms of the shared enquiry that has underpinned this chapter, action research has not been a linear process of knowing what to say and then saying it. We challenged ourselves to take a step, observe, reflect, and then adapt the words that appeared on the page. In this way the writing was a process of discovery (Richardson & St Pierre, 2008), allowing for continuous cycles of enquiry and change. This kind of enquiry fostered a dynamic interaction between thought and action, helping us carve new paths in the same way that rivers shape the landscape.

As we come to the end of our journey with you, we invite you to reflect on what becomes possible when we slow down and listen deeply, when we pause to consider meaning and purpose. When we realise that our healing is inextricably bound to the healing of the earth and all its living systems. As we close, we ask that you pause yourself to wonder, to ask and to act, guided by the knowledge that we are all part of this Patient Revolution.

References

Abram, D. (1995). *Ecopsychology: Restoring the earth, healing the mind* (T. Roszak, M. E. Gomes, & A. D Kanner, Eds.). Catapult.

Abram, D. (1997). *The spell of the sensuous.* Knopf Doubleday Publishing Group.

Akomolafe, B. The times are urgent: Let's slow down. https://www.bayoakomolafe.net/post/the-times-are-urgent-lets-slow-down

Benyus, J. M. (1997). *Biomimicry: Innovation inspired by nature.* Morrow.

Frank, A. W. (1995). *The wounded storyteller: Body, illness & ethics.* University of Chicago Press.

Heath, I. (2024). *John Berger: Ways of learning.* Oxford University Press.

Hine, D. (2023). *At work in the ruins: Finding our place in the time of science, climate change, pandemics and all the other emergencies.* Chelsea Green Publishing.

Launer, J. (2018). *Narrative-based practice in health and social care: Conversations inviting change.* Routledge.

Macy, J., & Brown, M. (2014). *Coming back to life: The updated guide to the work that reconnects* (2nd ed.). New Society Publishers.

Marsden, M. (2003). *The woven universe: Selected writings of Rev.* Māori Marsden.

May, K. (2023). *Enchantment: Reawakening wonder in an exhausted age.* Faber & Faber.

Macy, J., & Brown, M. Y. (2014). *Coming back to life: The updated guide to the work that reconnects* (2nd ed.). New Society Publishers.

Montori, V. (2020). *Why we revolt: A patient revolution for careful and kind care.* Rosetta Books.

Myat, J., Lewis, S., & Nicholls, C. (2024) *The cards.* https://www.thecards.org/the-cards

Pullman, P. *Philip Pullman quotes.* Retrieved 02/2025 from https://www.goodreads.com/author/quotes/3618.Philip_Pullman

Reason, P., & Bradbury, H. (2001). Introduction: Inquiry and participation in search of a world worthy of human aspiration. In P. Reason & H. Bradbury (Eds.), *Handbook of action research: Participative inquiry and practice* (pp. 1–14). Sage Publications.

Richardson, L., & St Pierre, E. (2008). A method of inquiry. In N. K. Denzin & Y. S. Lincoln (Eds.), *Handbook of qualitative research* (p. 473). Sage Publications.

Saunders, T. (2023). Rewiggling general practice. *BJGP Life.* https://bjgplife.com/rewiggling-general-practice/

Spiller, C., Barclay-Kerr, H., & Panoho, J. (2015). *Wayfinding leadership: Ground-breaking wisdom for developing leaders.* Huia Publishers.

Wallenburg, I., Weggelaar, A. M., & Bal, R. (2019). Walking the tightrope: How rebels "do" quality of care in healthcare organizations. *Journal of Health Organization and Management, 33*(7/8), 869–883. https://doi.org/10.1108/JHOM-10-2018-0305.

Yunkaporta, T. (2019). *Sand talk: How Indigenous thinking can save the world.* Harper Collins.

Index

For Product Safety Concerns and Information please contact our EU
representative GPSR@taylorandfrancis.com
Taylor & Francis Verlag GmbH, Kaufingerstraße 24, 80331 München, Germany

www.ingramcontent.com/pod-product-compliance
Lightning Source LLC
Chambersburg PA
CBHW050608280326
41932CB00016B/2959

9 7 8 1 0 3 2 8 3 2 1 6 6